The Mediterranean
Migraine Diet

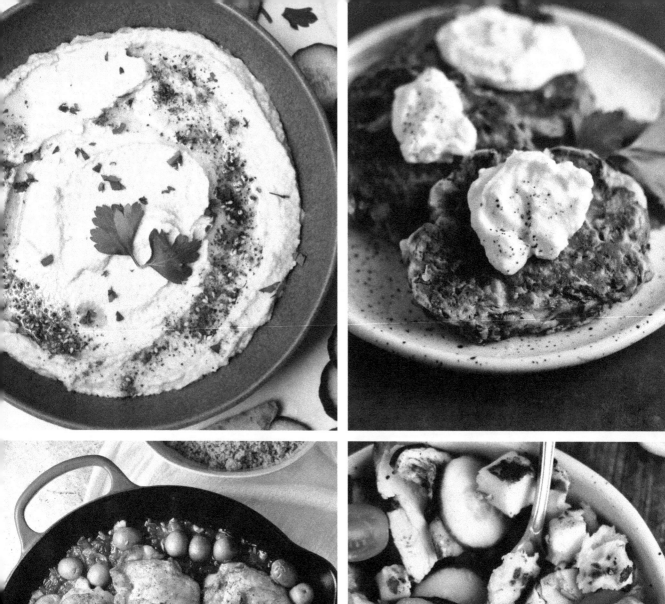
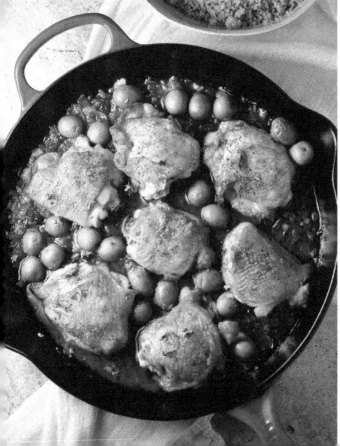
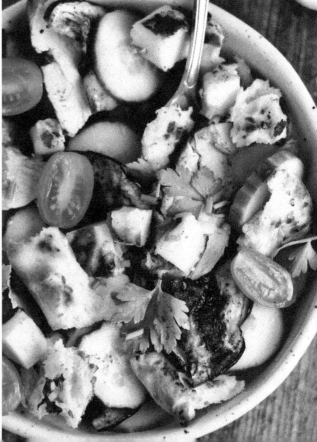

The Mediterranean Migraine Diet

A Science-Based Roadmap to Control Symptoms & Transform Brain Health

ALICIA WOLF & SHIN C. BEH, MD, FAAN, FAHS

WEST
MARGIN
PRESS

For those who feel lost, unheard, or unseen, this is for you.
May these recipes bring joy to your kitchen and better days ahead! —A.W.

To my patients, for whom I care, and from whom I learn. —S.B.

© 2022 by Alicia Wolf and Shin Beh, MD, FAAN, FAHS

Photographs by Alicia Wolf, except those by Angie Garcia on pages 6, 8, 12, 168, 204; marble Aon_Anda/Shutterstock; p. 18 Svetlana Lukienko/Shutterstock; p. 22 BigBlueStudio/Shutterstock; p. 23 Oleksandra Naumenko/Shutterstock; p. 24 Kiian Oksana/Shutterstock; p. 25 Fascinadora/Shutterstock; p. 26 masa44/Shutterstock; p. 29 nadianb/Shutterstock; p. 49 KatyaPulina/Shutterstock; p. 52 Mouse family/Shutterstock; p. 98 Netrun78/Shutterstock; p. 118 Mila Bond/Shutterstock; p. 190 White bear studio/Shutterstock; p. 210 Firanita/Shutterstock

Icons from the Noun Project: gluten-free by Stefan Parnarov; vegetarian by Karolina Bt; milk by Arthur Shlain; spatula by Nathan Driskell; stethoscope by Creative Mahira.

Edited by Jennifer Newens and Jessica Gould
Indexed by Elizabeth Parson

LS2022

Library of Congress Cataloging-in-Publication Data

Names: Wolf, Alicia, author. | Beh, Shin, author.
Title: The Mediterranean migraine diet : a science-based roadmap to control symptoms and transform brain health / Alicia Wolf & Shin Beh, M.D.
Description: [Berkeley, CA] : West Margin Press, [2022] | Includes bibliographical references and index. | Summary: "This cookbook features more than 70 delicious recipes plus photographs and dozens of helpful tips to help combat migraine symptoms by eating a Mediterranean-style diet"-- Provided by publisher.
Identifiers: LCCN 2022020348 (print) | LCCN 2022020349 (ebook) | ISBN 9781513134918 (paperback) | ISBN 9781513134925 (hardback) | ISBN 9781513134932 (ebook)
Subjects: LCSH: Migraine--Diet therapy. | Food allergy--Prevention.
Classification: LCC RC392 .W65 2022 (print) | LCC RC392 (ebook) | DDC 616.8/49120654--dc23/eng/20220601
LC record available at https://lccn.loc.gov/2022020348
LC ebook record available at https://lccn.loc.gov/2022020349

Published by West Margin Press®

WEST
MARGIN
PRESS

WestMarginPress.com

Proudly distributed by Ingram Publisher Services

WEST MARGIN PRESS
Publishing Director: Jennifer Newens
Marketing Manager: Alice Wertheimer
Project Specialist: Micaela Clark
Editor: Olivia Ngai
Design & Production: Rachel Lopez Metzger

CONTENTS

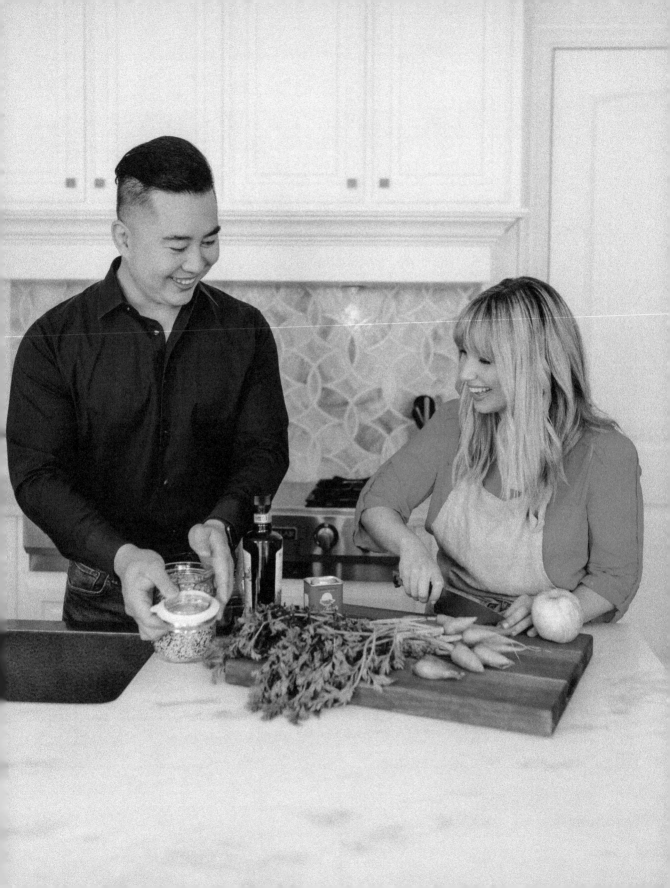

ABOUT THIS BOOK

As both a patient and a doctor who live with and treat migraine disorders, respectively, we know firsthand how important diet can be in treating migraine symptoms. Medication, supplements, monitoring sleep, managing stress, and focusing on hydration are also important, but we've both found that diet can be the final piece of the migraine puzzle that can help you achieve 100% symptom-free days.

But what does it mean to eat a healthy diet when you're living with migraine? Many doctors and online sources will simply supply you with a list of things to avoid and no real direction. That's why we decided to partner on a book that gives people living with migraine a science-based, yet practical approach to cooking and eating. Our Mediterranean migraine diet takes a style of eating that's proven to be optimal for brain health, and mixes in solid information on why certain foods might be a potential cause of migraine attacks more than others. Our philosophy doesn't label foods as good or bad but instead interprets their value by asking the question, "What is the best option for my brain?" It's truly a diet that can benefit everyone, and it's one that both doctors and patients can get behind. And, of course, it is delicious!

In this book you'll see substitutions for things like nuts, yogurt, tomatoes, citrus, or gluten and dairy, for those folks who find these to be personal triggers. This does not mean that these will be everyone's migraine triggers, or that they should be strictly avoided. They are just ideas for readers who might be sensitive.

We like to give people options! While it would be impossible to cater to everyone's individual triggers, we try to cover the most common ones.

In writing this book, we focused on balancing the flavors of the Mediterranean (featuring fruits, vegetables, grains, legumes, poultry, meat, and eggs that are great for our brains) with what is practical for a home cook living with migraine. While these recipes may not be a precise reflection of what you would be served if you visited the Mediterranean coast, they are optimized to make eating this way as delicious and easy as possible. If some ingredients seem unfamiliar or recipes seem intimidating, we encourage you to push outside your comfort zone a little bit. There's nothing quite like plating a meal that you never believed you could make, and to do it when you have a neurological disorder deserves a celebration. So, believe in yourself and lean into the joy of cooking. Put on some good music, take your time, make yourself a great mocktail, and celebrate the fact that following our Mediterranean migraine diet guidelines is improving your brain health one day at a time.

KEY TO THE RECIPES Look for these symbols throughout the book. They'll let you know who's writing as well as how you can adapt recipes to your personal needs.

NOTES FROM
ALICIA

NOTES FROM
DR. BEH

GLUTEN-FREE
OPTION

DAIRY-FREE
OPTION

PLANT-BASED
OPTION

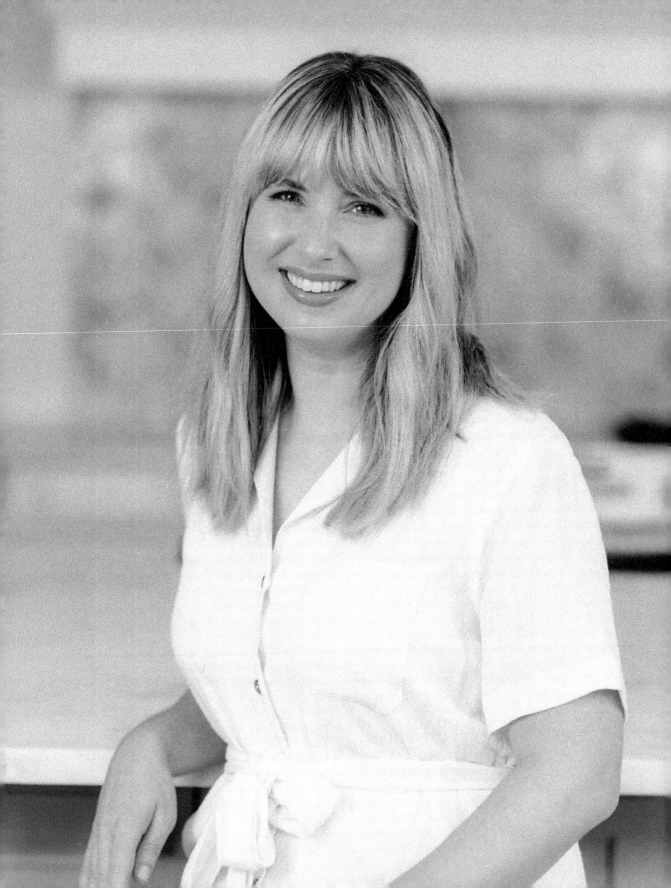

ALICIA'S STORY

My story begins with strange feelings of dizziness, like I was walking on marshmallows and my head was floating up in the clouds. I bounced from doctor to doctor for over six months without a diagnosis. My symptoms continued to escalate until one day I knew it was no longer safe for me to drive. I had just turned 30 and was newly married when vestibular migraine hit me like a ton of bricks.

Scary, vertigo-like symptoms began to appear—I felt like either I was moving, or the world around me was moving. Sometimes I felt completely detached from my body, as if my head would pop off and float away into the clouds. Grocery shopping became a painful experience where shelves would seemingly move on their own, and florescent lights felt like they burned my eyes. I never experienced head pain, as one would expect with migraine, only these very strange symptoms.

I continued to push for answers, leaving behind my family doctor to pursue one of the top ENTs in Dallas. After about a month of seeing him and all my tests coming back normal, he said he could no longer help me and suggested I see "The Dizzy Doctor," Dr. Shin Beh, a neurologist in the Dallas area. On the verge of losing my job, I put in a request to see Dr. Beh and was told he had a 7- to 8-month waiting list. Desperate, I called constantly to inquire about appointment cancellations.

In the meantime, I pursued other top professionals in Dallas who suspected I might be suffering from several awful things: MS, vestibular neuritis, a perilymph fistula that, if treated surgically, would leave me deaf. Many doctors just brushed me off as an anxious or depressed woman who was "stressed out" and claimed I wouldn't feel this way if I was better about managing my stress. I felt my life spiraling out of control. I was losing my job, my mind, and my identity.

Eventually, I found an ENT and perilymph fistula expert at the Mayo Clinic in Arizona. My husband drove me the 16 hours it took to get there because I was told by one of the physicians that I should not fly with a perilymph fistula. After two days of testing, the doctor walked in, looked me dead in the eyes, and said, "You don't have a perilymph fistula, you have migraine." I was floored. How could that be? I had never had a bad headache or anything I would classify as a "migraine" before (society has definitely engrained the concept that "migraine equals headache" in most people who have never experienced one). He explained to me that vestibular migraine was a less common type of migraine that can come with or without head pain, but presents mostly as dizziness, vertigo, and light sensitivity—in other words, all of my symptoms. Because this wasn't an area of expertise for him, he suggested I find a neurologist familiar with this vestibular migraine. What I didn't realize is there are very few of them!

It was that week I got the call from Dr. Beh's office he could squeeze me in. I brought my husband and my mom, and we sat in a row like three eager students, curious to see if this famous "dizzy doctor" would come to a similar conclusion. After evaluating all my notes and actually listening to what I said, he came to the same diagnosis—vestibular migraine.

NEW HOPE

With a diagnosis from two doctors I trusted, I felt more confident this was the answer I had been searching for. I decided I would accept this diagnosis and get on a treatment plan with Dr. Beh, doing everything I could to improve. In our first meeting,

I told him that we had planned on having a family soon and I leaned toward treatments that would not interfere with that. It was no problem for Dr. Beh! We worked on medication and supplement options together, as a team.

My healing did not happen overnight. And I remember very vividly in a follow-up appointment about six months later where I asked him, "Will I ever feel normal? Or is this my life forever?" I'll never forget how he looked me with complete confidence and said "Of course! Most of my patients I don't see anymore!" He went on to explain that his goal was to get patients on plans where either they were well-controlled with certain medications and they felt great again, or they had weaned off all medications and gone into remission. I tried to not take offense that he didn't actually want me as a patient forever, but instead saw it as a challenge. I was going to be one of those patients.

It took a lot of hard work and experimenting with different treatments, along with faith that I would be one of Dr. Beh's former patients one day. While I improved somewhat with supplements, medication, a predictable sleep schedule, therapy, and stress-relieving techniques, nearly two years later, changing my diet ended up being that last piece that got me to dizzy-free days.

After I lost my job due to this new chronic illness, and was depressed about so many things, my therapist suggested I focus on things I was passionate about, things that I loved doing. For me, that was cooking. I spent a lot of time dreaming of new recipes and trying different combinations in the kitchen, all the while searching for migraine-friendly products donning my migraine glasses and light-shielding ball cap.

I dreamed of creating a resource for people like myself, so that others wouldn't make the same mistakes I made as a migraine patient. That's how thedizzycook.com was born. I designed it to have the features of some of my favorite food blogs—with great recipes that everyone, with or without migraine, will love—coupled with stories about my personal journey with vestibular migraine to help others needing support. It turns out, my website was just what the migraine community needed.

Dr. Beh has supported me along the way. He's always open to doing interviews for my audience and answering the questions that very few other doctors can. And this is all information that never existed publicly just a mere six years ago. Having *The Dizzy Cook* site has allowed me to directly connect other patients like myself to his clinic, getting them the help that they desperately need. Not a day goes by that I don't connect a patient in need to "the dizzy doctor."

Even though I still have to work every day to keep my migraine trigger load down, most of my days are 100% symptom-free. Miraculously, this is even after going through IVF and having a very difficult pregnancy and postpartum period, which required revisiting new treatments and changing a few things around. Five years later I can now say I'm one of those patients Dr. Beh rarely sees anymore… that is, until we decided to write this book!

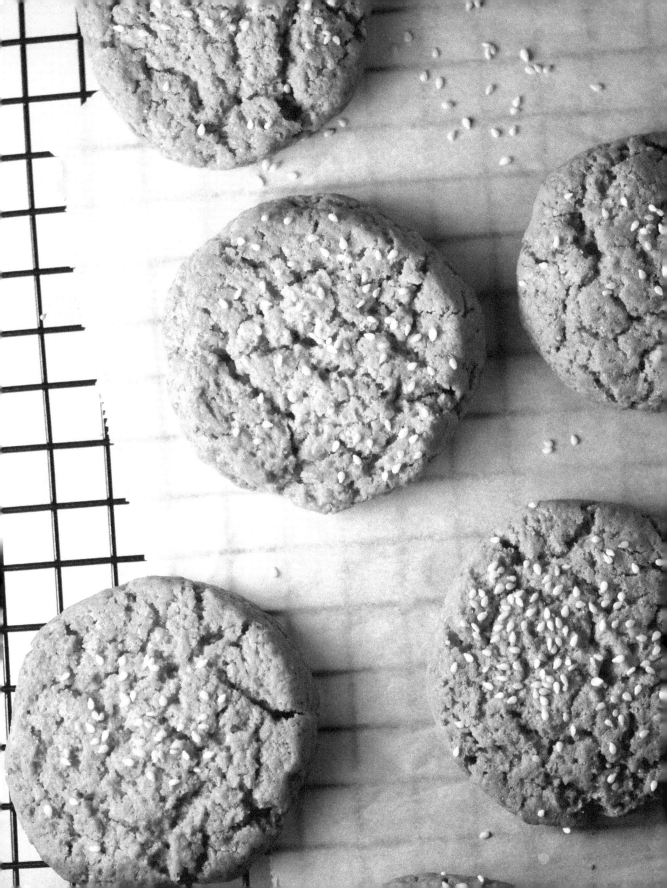

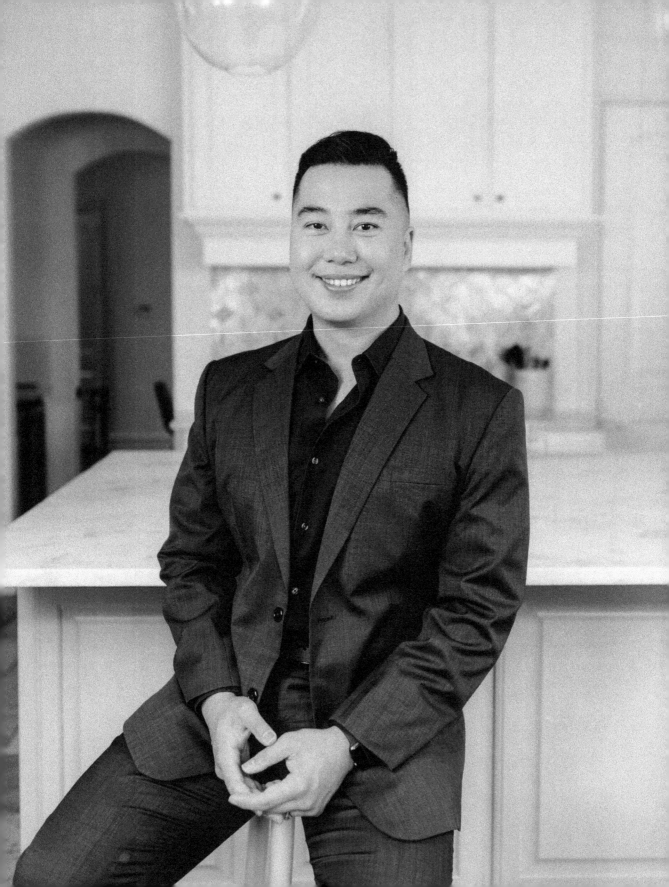

DR. BEH'S STORY

My journey into the world of oto-neurology (the subspecialty of neurology dealing with vertigo and dizziness) started in medical school. I recall my professor teaching about benign paroxysmal positional vertigo (BPPV), and how it could be easily diagnosed and treated at the bedside with a simple maneuver. When I was a visiting medical student in Singapore, the attending neurologists piqued my interest even more as they taught about vertigo, dizziness, nystagmus (repetitive, uncontrolled movements of the eyes), and the nuances of how to figure out which part of the vestibular system was affected. As a neurology resident, I was always fascinated by patients with vertigo and dizziness, especially when I saw how most medical specialties preferred not to deal with these symptoms. I embarked on a somewhat unorthodox three-center fellowship to train in multiple sclerosis, oto-neurology, and neuro-ophthalmology with some of the best teachers in the world at Johns Hopkins University, New York University, and UT Southwestern.

After I was recruited back to UT Southwestern as faculty, I initially divided my time between patients with multiple sclerosis and vestibular disorders. After a short time, I realized that the need for a neurologist who specialized in vestibular disorders was far greater, and focused my practice in that direction. I soon discovered that vestibular migraine affected a huge proportion of my patients, and I was astounded by how little we knew about the condition. Needless to say, that sparked my interest in learning more about vestibular migraine and exploring ways of treating it.

Much of my knowledge comes from my patients. They inform me about how this disorder manifests, which treatments work and which do not, and what side effects to watch out for. I distilled this experience into my book *Victory Over Vestibular Migraine* so the many patients who suffer from vestibular migraine, and their loved ones, would have a one-stop, comprehensive reference to learn about the symptoms of the disorder, as well as lifestyle and diet changes, nutraceuticals, and treatments to help them heal. I am truly humbled and touched by the many who tell me how much they have learned from my book.

In 2021, I founded The Beh Center for Vestibular & Migraine Disorders, a direct care practice to provide care to people with vertigo, dizziness, imbalance, and migraine disorders from all over the world.

I met Alicia as a patient early in my career. It has been remarkable to see how she has not only overcome vestibular migraine but has also transformed into an influencer who has raised so much awareness around this disorder and helped many people with their health journeys. It was so encouraging when she launched thedizzycook.com and *The Dizzy Cook*, resources that help so many people living with migraine. Our relationship is unique, and it has led us to collaborate on this new book to help people with migraine embrace a diet that not only avoids migraine triggers, but also has scientifically proven health benefits.

DIGGING INTO DIET

As a migraine patient, I remember feeling utterly confused when it came to changing my diet. I tried many things in an effort to diminish my 24/7 symptoms. It was not until I combined a migraine elimination diet by Johns Hopkins Dr. David Buchholz called *Heal Your Headache* with Dr. Beh's treatment plan that I began to see improvement.

A migraine elimination diet such as in the book *Heal Your Headache* can be tricky, especially if you have food allergies or sensitivities, but it's time well spent. The good news is that elimination diets are not meant to be a long-term way of eating. For example, once I successfully managed my symptoms through diet changes, and I had been feeling better for a while, I was able to reintroduce foods one by one to find my personal migraine food triggers. (Mine ended up being yogurt, caffeine, and nuts, which is why you will not see these in the recipes in this book.) Another thing I noticed is that moderation is key. For example, I cannot drink too much red wine or eat a lot of chocolate over several days, or they could trigger my symptoms. But they work for me as occasional treats.

As I incorporated more foods back into my diet, two principles really stuck with me. The first was to cook more at home. The second was to read labels and only bring home products with minimal ingredients. While cooking can be challenging as a chronic migraine patient, doing so helps you control what you eat because you know exactly what is going into your meals. You have more control over the sodium content, additives, and MSG—all of which can be personal migraine triggers in large amounts. Sodium, more specifically, can be a problem for those who have Meniere's disease in addition to migraine. For me, cooking at home leant a sense of accomplishment. Migraine had taken much from me—my career, my time (spent fighting with insurance companies and trying to find a doctor

who knew how to treat me), and my sense of wellbeing. Cooking at home doesn't need to be an everyday thing, but I hope that the suggestions in this book will also better guide your choices when eating out.

My first book, *The Dizzy Cook*, used the principles of the *Heal Your Headache* eating plan, also known as the Johns Hopkins migraine diet. If you are still in the process of figuring out your personal triggers, I recommend you read that book first. But if you are ready to branch out with new ingredients or want to learn how to eat to promote brain heath and lower inflammation, this book is the perfect choice. Alternatively, if you are overwhelmed by food lists and want to focus on healing recipes without the challenge and stress of a full elimination diet, this book is for you.

As you cook through this book, remember to celebrate the small and large wins along the way. Perhaps you finally conquered a fear of cooking a whole fish with my Roasted Branzino (page 158). Or you tried a new spice like za'atar or sumac. Branching outside of our comfort zones promotes healing along the way, opening ourselves up to new ideas and treatments. I know this from experience: If I had not been open to new things, I wouldn't have gone from being bedridden with constant symptoms to having 100% symptom-free days again—even after IVF treatments and postpartum complications. For that I have three main things to thank—Dr. Beh, cooking, and myself. Okay, and lots of magnesium too!

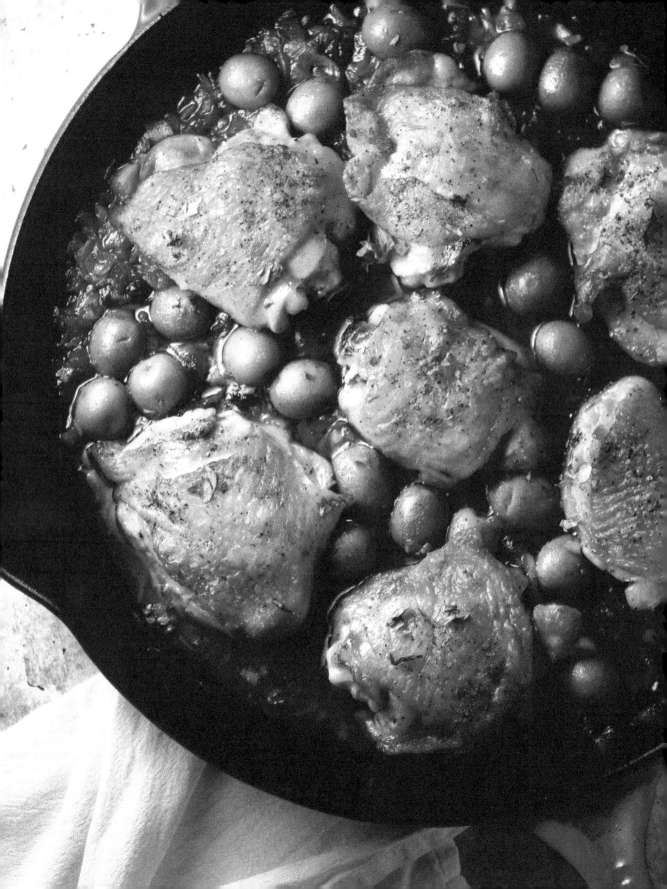

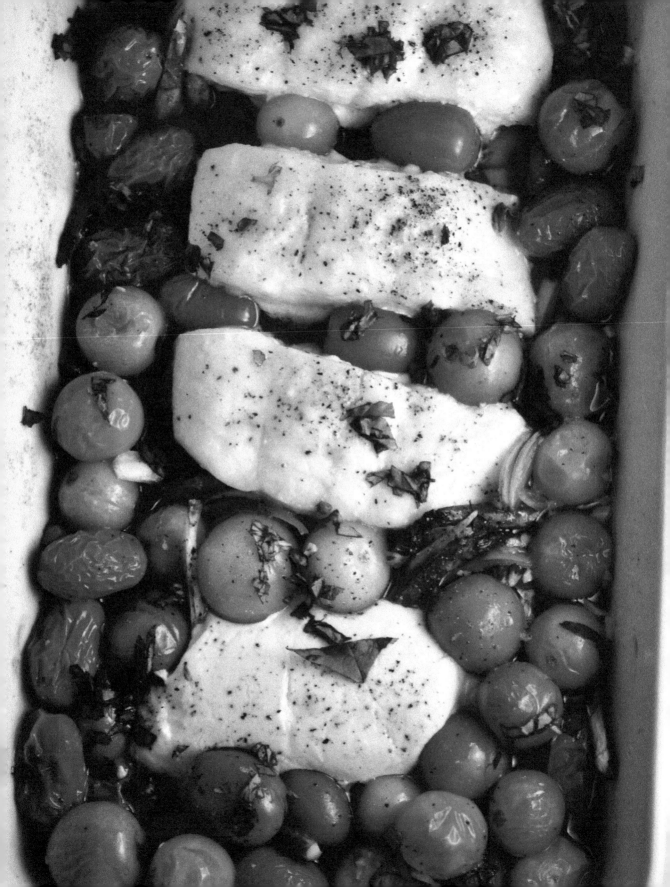

WHY CHOOSE THE MEDITERRANEAN DIET FOR MIGRAINE?

The Florentine diplomat and author Niccolò Machiavelli said that the true way to Paradise was to "learn the way to Hell in order to flee from it." Many migraine resources take a similar approach: warning people with migraine about various trigger foods to flee from. This approach is helpful but incomplete and leaves many wondering, "Well, what in the world can I eat?"

We wanted a resource that provides people with migraine a dietary roadmap to control symptoms and radically transform their health. While researching which dietary plan was best, we wanted a science- and evidence-based diet that could be adapted to the unique needs of people with migraine.

It is impossible to keep up with all the diets: the South Beach diet, paleo diet, MIND diet, low FODMAP, Atkins, keto, the DASH diet, vegan, flexitarian, alkaline diet, plant-based, the Zone diet, the blood-type diet, the Subway diet (remember Jared Fogle?), the Master Cleanse, the raw food diet, the Duke diet, Whole30, and more. How do we know which one is right? How do we know which one would help? Everyone claims to have evidence that their diet is effective. Every guru or doctor claims to hold the keys to the best diet for you. It is important that we weigh the scientific evidence for specific diets, especially as a migraine patient, and resist the temptation to jump on the latest fad.

WHAT IS THE MEDITERRANEAN DIET?

The Mediterranean diet has been practiced for generations and is backed by a strong body of scientific evidence. The cardiovascular benefits of the Mediterranean diet were first reported in the 1960s in the Seven Countries study. This famous study found that the Mediterranean diet, which was low in saturated fat and high in unsaturated fats, lowered the risk of cardiovascular disease [Keys, 1986]. This was a remarkable finding in an era when all dietary fat was considered bad. The HALE (Healthy Ageing–a Longitudinal study in Europe),

FINE (Finland, Italy, Netherlands Elderly), and SENECA (Survey in Europe on Nutrition in the Elderly) studies confirmed that the Mediterranean diet reduced the mortality rate by more than fifty percent. Many other studies have supported the numerous positive health benefits of this diet.

By contrast, the typical Western style of eating is a more recent product of the relentless industrialization of food. Instead of using fresh, sustainable ingredients, it focuses on products that are cheap and quick to manufacture, last for a long time, and induce a brief feeling of pleasure in our brains. A typical Western diet is loaded with sugar, refined carbohydrates, unhealthy amounts of omega-6 fatty acids, saturated fats, artificial trans fats, and additives with long, unpronounceable names. It is devoid of fiber, complex carbohydrates, bioactive polyphenols, omega-3 fatty acids, mono-unsaturated and polyunsaturated fats, vitamin C, riboflavin, magnesium, and folate. The epidemic of non-communicable lifestyle diseases like obesity, diabetes, hypertension, stroke, neurodegenerative diseases, cancers, depression, anxiety, and auto-immune diseases testify to how detrimental such a diet is to our health.

When my patients ask me if there is a diet to control migraine symptoms, I talk to them about elimination diets, like *Heal Your Headache*. But when they are feeling better and want a more sustainable eating plan, I tell them that there is no "ultimate" supplement that will miraculously make you feel better or prolong your life. Transforming one's diet

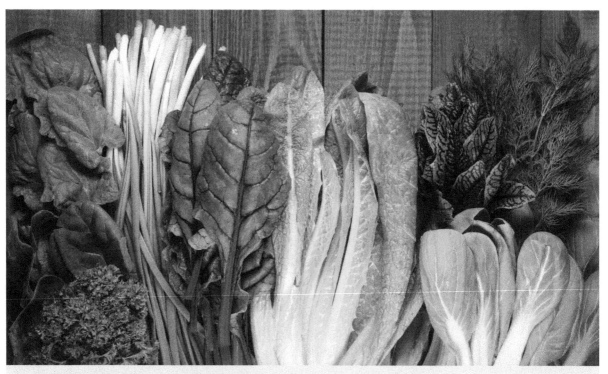

MEDITERRANEAN DIET GUIDELINES

The ten key guidelines of the Mediterranean diet are:

1 Use olive oil (especially EVOO, extra virgin olive oil) as the main fat source. Aim to consume at least 4 tablespoons of olive oil per day.

2 Always eat fresh and minimally processed foods.

3 Eat plenty of fruits and vegetables.

4 Eat whole-grain products.

5 Make fish and poultry the primary protein source.

6 Consume dairy products in moderation.

7 Consume red meat in small amounts.

8 Limit saturated fat consumption.

9 Always avoid artificial trans fats.

10 Enjoy red wine in moderation, with one meal a day.

It is never too late to change your diet and transform your health. Many studies prove that switching from an average unhealthy Western diet to the Mediterranean diet results in significant, tangible health benefits. In this book, we've taken things a step further: We've taken advantage of all the health benefits of the Mediterranean diet and adapted it to the needs of people with migraine. The antioxidant and anti-inflammatory properties of the Mediterranean diet are ideal for those who suffer from this debilitating neurological condition. The focus on fresh, flavorful foods, and the minimal use of processed, highly refined ingredients promote a healthier internal physiologic environment, which in turn helps the migraine brain.

and health is a lifelong journey. Therefore, a logical, well-supported, and sustainable dietary approach is crucial. The Mediterranean diet takes a well-balanced, evidence-based, and (most important of all) flavorful approach to fresh, healthy foods that can be sustained over a lifetime, and does not just focus on depriving yourself. It also features many brain-healthy ingredients that can help a migraine patient have a better quality of life for the long run.

The scientifically proven benefits of the Mediterranean diet can be attributed to a high content of antioxidants, anti-inflammatory agents, bioactive polyphenols, fiber, and healthy fats, which consist of monounsaturated fatty acids (MUFAs) and polyunsaturated fats (PUFAs). The Mediterranean diet also contains few refined carbohydrates (like sugar and white flour) and unhealthy fats (saturated animal fats and trans fats). The higher omega-3 fatty acid intake of the Mediterranean diet reduces inflammatory processes; the higher omega-6 fatty acid content of a typical Western diet, on the other hand, favors a more inflammatory state. The higher fiber and polyphenol content of the Mediterranean diet creates a healthier and more diverse gut microbiome, which can also have a positive effect on the brain.

In addition to lowering inflammation and offering brain health benefits, the following characteristics are believed to contribute to the proven benefits of the Mediterranean diet:

- Lowering cancer risk. The Mediterranean diet can lower the risk of various cancers, including prostate, breast, and colorectal cancer.

- Promoting healthy weight. The Mediterranean diet helps maintain healthy body weight and reduces obesity. Switching from a typical American diet to the Mediterranean diet results in improved weight control, even without changing caloric intake [Jaacks, 2018]. It is more effective than a low-fat diet at keeping the pounds off as well.

- Improving cardiovascular health. The landmark Spanish study Prevencion con Dieta Mediterranea (PREDIMED) proved that the Mediterranean diet cuts the risk for heart disease and stroke, and substantially reduces the risk of developing diabetes and promotes healthy blood pressure.

- Enhancing the mood. Proving that what we eat affects how we feel, several studies show that the Mediterranean diet enhances the mood and a sense of well-being and reduces the risk of depression (a common complaint among migraine patients).

- Improving cognitive abilities. In human and animal studies, olive oil has been shown to improve learning ability and the formation of synapses. Furthermore, the Mediterranean diet decreases the risk for neurodegenerative diseases like Parkinson's disease and dementia.

- Reducing autoimmune disease activity. For example, inflammatory bowel disease, and chronic hives.

According to the United Nations Educational, Scientific, and Cultural Organization (UNESCO), the Mediterranean diet is part of the intangible cultural heritage of Greece, Italy, Spain, Cyprus, Croatia, Portugal, and Morocco. It has been practiced and handed down over thousands of years by the people of the region.

TRANS FATS

Trans fats are manufactured fats that are used to prolong the shelf life of food products. They are not metabolized by the body, but instead float around in the blood stream, triggering inflammation, promoting atherosclerosis, and increasing cancer risk. Examples of trans fats include margarine and traditional vegetable shortening. When you are shopping, look at the ingredient list; if it states "hydrogenated," or "partially hydrogenated" vegetable oil or fats, toss it back on the shelf. Fried foods, especially fast food, often harbor large amounts of trans fats.

MIGRAINE FOOD TRIGGERS

 There are many resources that discuss migraine food triggers in detail. We will keep this chapter succinct and highlight certain important points. Each person has their unique food triggers, and not all foods known to trigger migraine attacks will do so in every single person with migraine. Some foods trigger migraine in a significant number of people. The list of triggers should thus be used as guide, and not as a list of forbidden foods.

CAFFEINE As a rule, I advise my patients not to consume more than the equivalent of one to two cups (8 to 16 ounces) of coffee a day. In migraine studies, more than two cups per day causes a worsening of migraine frequency. Furthermore, excessive caffeine intake can exacerbate anxiety, and causes dehydration, which in and of itself is a migraine trigger.

CHOCOLATE For a long time, chocolate has been a suspected migraine trigger. While there is mixed scientific evidence, there are several chemical compounds in chocolate that can trigger migraine, including caffeine, tyramine, phenylalanine, and naturally occurring nitrates. Furthermore, commercially sold chocolate products often contain many other additives, including sugar (lots of it), flavoring, preservatives, and coloring.

TYRAMINE Tyramine is the by-product of the breakdown of tyrosine, an amino acid found in many foods. Tyramine is a known migraine trigger, and foods containing high levels of tyramine are often implicated in migraine attacks. As a guideline, the tyramine content of foods increases during the aging, curing, fermentation, or ripening process. Fresh or frozen foods contain little tyramine. Canning foods also halts tyramine growth, so it's generally safe to eat things like canned tuna.

Some fresh food like citrus, figs, coconuts, dates, pineapple, fava beans, and broad beans have naturally higher levels of tyramine. Nuts are a rich source of monounsaturated and polyunsaturated fatty acids but have levels of tyramine that may trigger migraine attacks in some. Many condiments that enhance flavor, including soy and fish sauce, contain high levels of tyramine.

MONOSODIUM GLUTAMATE (MSG) MSG adds to the umami (savory) taste of food. It is found naturally in many foods, including tomatoes, seaweed, and cheese. In 1908, Japanese biochemist Kikunae Ikeda isolated MSG as the compound responsible for the savory taste of seaweed used in many Japanese dishes. It is commonly added to commercially produced food products, like chips, bouillon, and soups, as a flavor enhancer. In small amounts, it is generally safe, but some people with migraine may be more sensitive to its migraine-triggering effects.

NITRATES/NITRITES & SULFITES These are food additives that prolong the shelf-life and appearance of food. Nitrates/nitrites are often used in processed or cured meats, like bacon, sausage, ham, and lunchmeats. Besides being known migraine triggers, nitrite in processed meats can react with heat to produce nitrosamines, which are toxic cancer-causing substances. Sulfites are used in dried, canned, or bottled fruit and vegetable products.

A PATIENT'S PERSPECTIVE ON RED WINE

I've always appreciated the process of winemaking and discovering great quality wines. In the past, I stuck with big name brands. And then I developed my migraine disorder and stopped drinking wine. After I started to feel better, one of my first trips was to Santa Ynez and Buellton in California, made famous by the movie *Sideways*. I remember being so nervous to try red wine again, especially since it gets some pretty bad press in the migraine community. What I learned from these smaller winemakers was that finding wineries with sustainable practices can make a huge difference in how your body tolerates the wine.

If wine ingredients were printed on a label, you might see a lot of additives and flavorings in addition to just grapes. One example of this is sulfites, which are a known migraine trigger. Sulfites are a natural biproduct of fermentation, and some wineries add additional sulfites to preserve the wine (it's a myth that organic wines are sulfite-free). However, different wines can have more or less sulfites depending on the grapes and how they are processed. But sulfites aren't the only culprit in wine for triggering migraine. Truly, it depends on how sensitive you are to the alcohol or to certain grapes, if the wine has any additives, or the fermentation process. Here are a few tips I've picked up that have helped me re-introduce wine to my diet in moderation.

- Choose small-batch wineries that focus on sustainable practices. Generally, these wineries are letting the grapes speak for themselves without adding flavorings or manipulating the wine. They also tend to use higher quality grapes and cut out any rot, naturally reducing the biogenic amine content, which some people are sensitive to.
- Lighter reds like pinot noir or merlot tend to be better tolerated than heavier wines such as cabernet sauvignon. Using PureWine's Wand™ wine purifier can also help reduce the histamine and sulfite content in any wine you choose.
- Before consuming wine, review your trigger load. I tend to have a higher migraine threshold when I'm on vacation and can easily tolerate a glass of wine, versus when I'm at home and more stressed out with my day-to-day activities. Perhaps this plays a part when people say they tolerate wines they had in Italy or France better than those they drink at home!

RED WINE Most of us are familiar with the beautiful fatty decadence of French food. Despite a high dietary saturated fat intake, the mortality rate among the French is three times lower than that of other industrialized countries. This is called the French paradox, and is believed to be due to the Mediterranean diet, which includes regular moderate red wine consumption. The cardiovascular benefits of red wine come from its rich content of polyphenols. The key word here is *moderate*—one drink a day with a meal. Imbibing more than that increases the risk of mortality.

Red wine has many health benefits. However, it also contains a variety of chemical compounds—histamine, sulfites, phenylethylamine, prostaglandins, tyramine, phenolic flavonoids, and tannins—which are implicated as potential migraine triggers. Red wine consumption is thus generally not advisable for those with migraine. However, if red wine is not one of your personal triggers, you can consume it in moderate quantities.

CURATING A MIGRAINE-FRIENDLY PANTRY

The best way to start transitioning your diet to be more migraine-friendly is to begin with the pantry. When I was struggling with chronic vestibular migraine and started to change what I was eating, I was astonished by the number of items in my pantry that contained lots of potential trigger foods—chips with all kinds of seasonings; sauces, condiments, and dressings with lots of preservatives; MSG; or aged vinegars and broths that also contained hidden glutamate. Here are some tips on what to look for when shopping.

BREAD I find that my local bakery or grocery store bakery is the best bet for good bread. Whole wheat or seeded breads are a favorite. Some migraine patients are triggered by fresh yeast. If this is the case for you, just wait a day to consume any bakery yeast breads or freeze them to use later. Pre-packaged breads can also work well, like Dave's Killer Bread and Pepperidge Farm Whole Wheat. For buns, I love Martin's Potato Buns, often found at Target, or whole wheat buns from a local bakery. For gluten-free, Free Bread makes a great loaf.

As for pizza crusts or flatbreads, I like to use pita (or even naan) as a base and create personal pizzas. This avoids any yeast sensitivities and cuts down the effort of making a crust from scratch. Another option is to use premade cauliflower crusts, especially if you want some extra vegetables! Watch out for aged cheese with those crusts.

BROTH AND STOCK If I'm buying store-bought broth and stock, I almost always choose a low-sodium vegetable broth. This is because I can avoid a high glutamate content, since many brands add "natural chicken flavor" or "natural beef flavor" to packaged varieties. If you're sensitive to tyramine and glutamate, it's best to avoid bone broth. The gelatinous texture from collagen increases as the broth is simmered, and although it yields many health benefits, it can be a sneaky migraine trigger. I discovered this the hard way when I added collagen peptides to my daily smoothie, which was

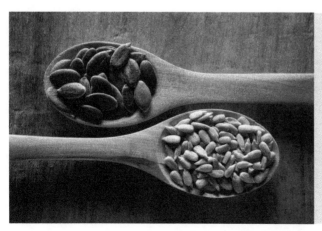

ABOUT SEEDS

Seeds are nutrient-packed superfoods that should be part of your diet. Sesame seeds are important in Mediterranean cuisine and are rich in a polyphenol called sesamin. Pumpkin and sunflower seeds are great sources of fiber, monounsaturated fats, and vitamin E. Flax and chia seeds are rich in omega-3 fatty acids, polyphenols, and fiber.

causing me a low level of dizziness that I couldn't quite pinpoint for a long time.

Making your own broth is easy and inexpensive with an Instant Pot. The whole process takes 20 to 40 minutes and can use up vegetable scraps, herbs, garlic, and the bones from your leftover rotisserie chicken. Without the long simmer time, making stock in an Instant Pot is a great method for those who are tyramine and histamine sensitive. You can find recipes for broth in my first book, *The Dizzy Cook.*

CONDIMENTS Prepared mayonnaise is a great condiment to have on hand, as making your own, although delicious, can be time consuming. I recommend looking for a prepared mayonnaise with olive oil or avocado oil as the base. With sunflower and soybean oil, which are high in omega-6 fatty acids, you want to balance it with omega-3s, which the recipes in this book do! A personal favorite of mine

is Sir Kensington's, which has straightforward ingredients. Other good brands include Spectrum Olive Oil Mayonnaise, Primal Kitchen, and Chosen Foods Avocado Oil. In general, try to avoid brands with "natural flavors" or modified food starches.

That said, the best mayonnaise to use would be homemade. It is easier to make than you probably think and there are plenty of recipes online. All you need are eggs, olive oil, vinegar or lemon, and salt and pepper. Pasteurized eggs make the process a little easier, but it's easy to clean the shells at home too. Two important factors for making homemade mayo are to start with a room temperature egg and use a high-speed food processor or an immersion blender. If oil is added too quickly to the mixture, everything will fall apart. If you're trying to eat more plant-based foods, I've included a recipe for chickpea mayonnaise on page 134, which has a wonderful flavor and lush texture.

With Dijon or other types of mustard, look out for sulfites which are often included, especially if the product contains wine. Annie's Dijon is a good one that I use often, but there are other brands out there.

CRACKERS As a Mediterranean diet suggests eating whole grains whenever possible, look for whole-wheat or whole-grain crackers such as original or sea salt Triscuits. For a gluten-free cracker, I love Crunchmasters Sea Salt, which also contain flax and sesame seeds. When shopping for crackers, be sure to check the label for any flavorings that might be a trigger; I find it's often best to go with plain crackers.

FLOUR All-purpose flour is generally migraine-friendly, but some people can be sensitive to malted barley, which is in many brands. If you suspect this is an issue for you, I recommend Bob's Red Mill Unbleached Organic White All-Purpose Flour, Arrowhead Mills Organic White

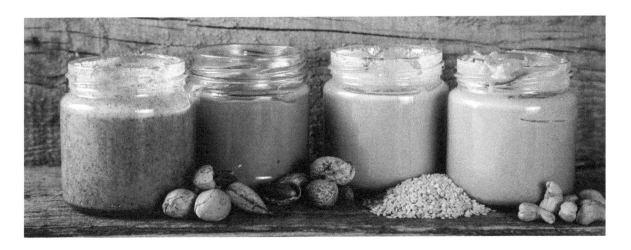

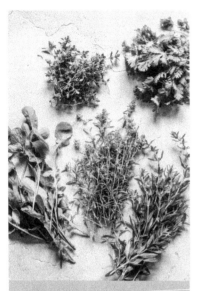

ABOUT HERBS & SPICES

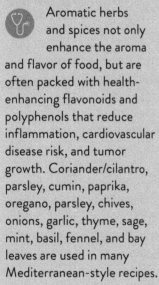

Aromatic herbs and spices not only enhance the aroma and flavor of food, but are often packed with health-enhancing flavonoids and polyphenols that reduce inflammation, cardiovascular disease risk, and tumor growth. Coriander/cilantro, parsley, cumin, paprika, oregano, parsley, chives, onions, garlic, thyme, sage, mint, basil, fennel, and bay leaves are used in many Mediterranean-style recipes.

Flour, White Wings La Paloma All-Purpose Flour, and Gold Medal All-Purpose Flour.

While gluten is not a general migraine trigger, it can be for those who have a gluten intolerance or sensitivity. You'll see edits within the recipes for modifying a recipe to be gluten-free. I find Bob's Red Mill 1:1 Gluten Free All-Purpose Flour works great for baking. To thicken sauces, cornstarch or arrowroot powder work very well.

JUICE Tart cherry juice and pomegranate juice, as well as apple and pear juice, are the ones I use most often in cooking. Check the ingredients to make sure you're just getting juice and no added sugars or flavors. RW Knudsen juices are widely available and sugar-free.

NUT AND SEED BUTTERS Nuts are an incredibly healthy snack option, and nut butters are widely available these days. However, I know that many people find nuts to be a personal migraine trigger, myself included. For these recipes, feel free to add in your favorite nuts if they're not an issue for you.

An alternative to nut butters is seed butters, which I find to be delicious. I reach for sunflower seed butter over peanut butter often! I like to use brands that are unsweetened and very lightly salted. They vary a lot in flavor, so test a few to find your favorite.

Pumpkin seed butter and watermelon seed butter are two seed butters that should not be missed. 88 Acres has a pumpkin seed butter that's wonderful on toast or in smoothies, and their watermelon seed butter works as an aioli substitute, tahini substitute, or even a vegan queso.

Tahini, sesame seed paste, makes wonderful dressings and sauces and can be used to add creaminess to a dish without the addition of dairy. Tahini has a distinct nutty flavor that works well with honey, in hummus recipes, or drizzled on roasted vegetables.

OIL AND BUTTER In general, cooking oils should be fine to use because they are so processed that personal triggers like peanuts, soy, or avocado tend to not be an issue. However, when focusing on a Mediterranean way of eating, unsaturated oils such as olive oil, nut oils, and flax seed oil are best to use for cooking.

Extra-virgin olive oil (EVOO) is what we use for the recipes in this book. This means the oil is unrefined, at its flavorful best, and not treated with heat. Olive oil can go rancid a lot faster than you might expect, so you want to be wary of giant bulk bottles unless you're using lots of it often. Keeping it in a cool dark place will help prevent rancidity—therefore many bottles are tinted dark to protect it from the light. Check the expiration date on the EVOO you already have in the pantry!

I like to choose two olive oils: one that's a good everyday brand, which I'll pick up at Trader Joe's, Lucini, or California Olive Ranch. This can be used as the base for most recipes. For the second, I'll keep a fun "fancy" bottle with stronger flavors to use as a drizzle on roasted or grilled vegetables, simple salads, or even vanilla ice cream! I like to pick one up on vacation—Spain, Italy, and Greece are great places to find delicious olive oil. However, you don't have to travel far—just find a local store that will let you taste a few and pick out a favorite.

Although not often used in Mediterranean cooking, butter was also used in the 2021 study that researched omega-3 and omega-6 fatty acids for migraine reduction. Participants that saw a reduction in attacks ate butter, extra-virgin olive oil, and macadamia nut oil. Although the Mediterranean diet utilizes butter sparingly, when buying it, be sure the ingredients are cream and salt (if buying salted), and nothing else. Some brands will add "natural flavor," which can be a potential source of glutamate and, thus, a migraine trigger. Kerrygold is a favorite that is widely available, but check your local store for a house brand that might be less expensive.

OLIVES There is some debate over whether olives are a migraine trigger and over my years of advocating, I have not noticed them to be a common issue. What

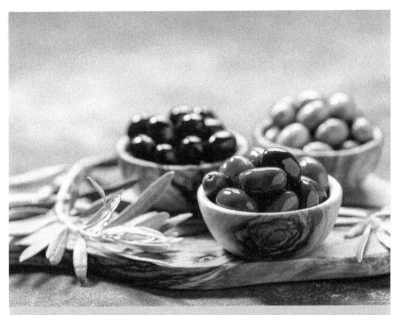

ABOUT OLIVES

Olive trees were cultivated in the Mediterranean regions 7,000 years ago. Olive oil, as discussed earlier, is an amazing superfood packed with monounsaturated fatty acids and polyphenols. This superfood is one of the main reasons the Mediterranean diet is associated with so many health benefits, including cutting the risk of cardiovascular disease, obesity, diabetes, stroke, and cancer.

Olive oil is not the only healthy derivative from olive fruits. Olives are also a good source of fiber, iron, copper, and antioxidants. Table olives can be categorized according to the degree of ripeness: green olives, semi-ripe olives (the skin turning from green to shades of red or brown), and black (ripe) olives. Raw olives are naturally bitter and have to be cured or fermented to make them palatable. This process increases the tyramine content of olive fruits, which can trigger migraine.

seems to help my readers who are sensitive to olives tolerate them better is to buy whole olives, which are less processed than pitted, and olives that are packed in water versus a brine or vinegar. Therefore, I suggest whole olives in all the recipes. Another trick is to try green olives over black olives, as green olives are picked before they are ripe. I love Castelvetrano olives, which have a light and buttery flavor and don't go through a fermentation process. Instead, they are bathed in a water and lye solution over the course of two weeks to remove the bitterness.

PASTA Any type of pasta is usually very migraine-friendly, and this is one thing you don't have to make at home! These recipes work equally well with semolina or whole-wheat pasta. You could also use chickpea pasta, but note that it tends to have a stronger flavor. Watch for added pea protein in chickpea pasta, which can be a trigger for some who are MSG-sensitive. Olo has one with very simple ingredients.

For gluten-free pasta, one of my favorite brands is Jovial, which tends to have the best texture and taste and it comes in a variety of shapes and sizes. They even have a cassava orzo!

SEASONINGS Most spices are well-tolerated for people with migraine, and many, such as cinnamon, turmeric, and ginger, offer health benefits. A few things to look out for come down to personal sensitivities, like cocoa powder or onion powder, which can be common in chili powder mixes. Don't worry about silicone dioxide. It's simply an anti-caking agent that helps prevent clumping. Also, don't worry about paying a higher price for organic—a varied spice drawer is more important!

Some Mediterranean spices I use in this book include sumac and za'atar. Sumac has a lovely tangy flavor that pairs well with chicken, hummus, and fish. Za'atar is a blend of cumin, sesame seeds, and sumac, which gives it a bright but earthy flavor. It pairs amazingly with roasted and grilled meat, or pretty much any vegetable. Although these two spices are less common in the U.S., they're increasingly becoming more widely available. Look for them in the bulk spice section of a well-stocked grocery store or from an online source.

SPARKLING WATER Sparkling water mixed with fruit juices or fresh fruit can make a great substitute for those struggling to let go of sugary soda drinks. I find Topo Chico to be the best for mixing because it stays fizzy even when you add juice.

VINEGAR Red and white wine vinegars are recommended on a traditional Mediterranean diet, but they contain sulfites, which can be troublesome for migraine patients. I've considered using a PureWine Wine Wand™ on aged vinegar to remove the sulfites before cooking, especially when using large amounts. But I find it easiest to cook with distilled white vinegar or lemon juice.

Distilled white vinegar, AKA acetic acid, is wonderful for a multitude of kitchen tasks. From cleaning fruits, vegetables, and countertops, to making a quick homemade buttermilk or poaching the perfect egg—it's my favorite vinegar! In the U.S., stores will often carry their own brand name; Heinz is also a common one. In other parts of the world, look for "white vinegar."

OMEGA-6 FATTY ACIDS

Omega-6 fatty acids are a family of polyunsaturated fatty acids, which are the precursors to pro-inflammatory proteins (e.g., eicosanoids, leukotrienes). The main dietary source of omega-6 fatty acids is vegetable oil, which is used in a wide variety of processed foods (e.g., mayonnaise) and in fried fast foods. A diet high in omega-6 fatty acids is pro-inflammatory, and can promote atherosclerosis, and aggravate autoimmune and inflammatory diseases.

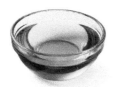

ABOUT OLIVE OIL

Look for good quality extra-virgin olive oil, which should have at least 73% oleic acid and less than 10% linoleic acid, for an oleic to linoleic acid ratio greater than 7.

OTHER INGREDIENT NOTES

 The following are some common ingredients I use and details on where to find them, what to look for, and how they can be modified for certain recipes and special diets.

CITRUS Although not a common migraine trigger, citrus does increase symptoms for a few. It's one of the ingredients that is recommended to avoid on a migraine elimination diet because large amounts can be high in tyramine. In this book I use very small amounts to complement other flavors, but I also give edits to replace citrus with white vinegar or other ingredients. If citrus is not something that you notice is a personal issue for you, feel free to use either option in the recipe.

CHEESE Cheese is eaten regularly in low to moderate amounts in a traditional Mediterranean diet, and dairy products can be great for brain health, assuming there is no sensitivity or intolerance. However, cheese can be a natural source of tyramine, which increases as a cheese ages. Parmesan is high in both tyramine and glutamate, so I tend not to use it. Instead, my recipes focus on using fresh, young cheeses like soft goat cheese, feta (un-aged), halloumi, mozzarella, burrata, good American cheese, cream cheese, mascarpone, ricotta, and cottage cheese.

For soft cheeses like ricotta or cream cheese, look for brands without carrageenan, an extract from red seaweed that is used as a thickener or gelling agent. Not only can it be a common migraine trigger, but it also makes ricotta cheese very gritty. Ricottas without added thickeners like Calabro, Liuzzi, and BelGiosio are only slightly more expensive than other varieties, but they have a huge difference in both flavor and texture.

Common Mediterranean cheeses like halloumi and feta tend to have high sodium levels, which can be a factor in triggering symptoms for some patients with Meniere's disease (which can be comorbid with vestibular migraine). Meniere's patients need to restrict their sodium intake. In these recipes, I recommend substituting a soft goat cheese (chevre) for these saltier cheeses; it is very low in sodium by comparison.

As is typical in the Mediterranean diet, cheese in these recipes is meant to highlight existing flavors, and not be the star of the show. For some recipes, you can leave it out entirely and still have a very delicious dish. For

others, you can try vegan cheese substitutes, but I recommend being cautious. Nutritional yeast and packaged vegan cheeses tend to be extremely high in glutamate, so if you're sensitive to MSG it's something to watch out for. If you're interested in a vegan cheese substitute and can tolerate glutamate in higher amounts, the most well tolerated seems to be Violife feta substitute.

Look at Costco, Trader Joe's, and Aldi for the best deals on cheese. It makes a wonderful snack, especially topped with fresh herbs, a little olive oil or honey.

DAIRY Butter and milk are good places to spend a little more money when it comes to choosing high quality products. I've already mentioned butter on page 25. For milk, organic, grass-fed milk will always be a tastier option, but choose what is most affordable for you. For the recipes in this book, I sometimes make preferred suggestions. Lower-fat milks tend to curdle much easier than whole milk, which makes them difficult to use in soups that need to be simmered. In that case, I like to choose a splash of heavy cream. This way of eating limits the

FATTY ACIDS

 Butter and ghee contain high amounts of saturated fatty acids, which can increase the risk of atherosclerosis. The Mediterranean diet consists of more polyunsaturated and monounsaturated fatty acids, which are healthier, and as such, we recommend limiting the use of butter and ghee.

amount of cream and butter used but does not necessarily eliminate it. Remember: everything in moderation!

For those who are lactose and casein sensitive, try ghee, also known as clarified butter. This is butter that has been simmered and separated from the milk solids so that only the pure butterfat remains. Ghee's flavor is a little nuttier than that of butter, but it also has a higher smoke point and can be heated to higher temperatures without burning.

Also dairy free is duck fat (leftover from Seared Duck with Cherry Sauce—page 188—or store-bought). I use it as a butter substitute in savory breakfast recipes, for roasted potatoes, in stews, or anywhere I want a deep, almost bacon-like flavor. Duck fat also contains a balanced amount of omega 3s to omega 6s.

HERBS If you use a lot of fresh herbs, consider planting a mini herb garden. Mint, basil (except in the winter), thyme, and rosemary grow very well and are commonly used throughout the Mediterranean region. Keeping a few of these plants in your backyard or on a windowsill can save you a lot of money over time—plus you always have them on hand. Storing fresh herbs in a water glass in the refrigerator can make them last much longer than they normally would. I have parsley that looks amazing even after two weeks!

When purchasing dried oregano, pass over bottles labeled "Mexican oregano" and instead look for options labeled "oregano" or "Mediterranean oregano," which will be more complimentary to these flavors.

ONIONS & SHALLOTS You may notice I don't use regular onions in any recipes. After cooking for a migraine elimination diet for so long, which calls for eliminating them, I found that I much prefer the flavor of shallots in recipes. In the cooking classes I've taken, this sentiment is often echoed because shallots are actually very closely related to garlic. The flavor is subtle and refined. Shallots also contain a higher amount of fiber and essential minerals like vitamin B6. While you could substitute onion for shallots in these recipes, keep in mind it will change the flavor of the final dish, with the onion flavor more pronounced.

SPINACH This is a wonderful, nutrient-packed green that I love to use in recipes. However, for those who are extremely sensitive to histamine, you can replace it in any of these recipes with lower-histamine greens like kale, arugula, or romaine. I recommend using kale in any soups or for the Ricotta Kale Fritters on page 68, and romaine and arugula in salads or as sandwich toppings.

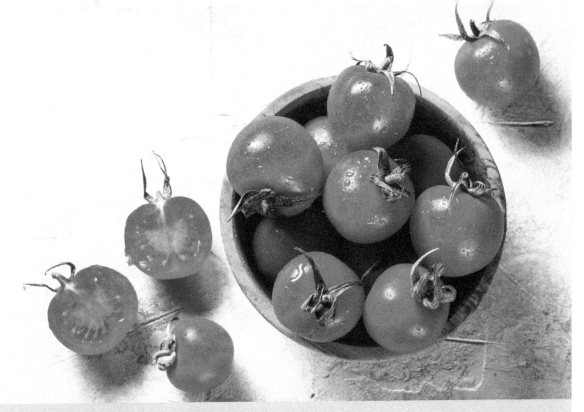

ABOUT TOMATOES

Tomatoes are fruits (not vegetables) that originate from Mexico but were spread around the world following Spanish colonization. Fresh tomato is used in many Mediterranean dishes. Tomatoes are rich in carotenoids (mainly lycopene and beta-carotene), a variety of polyphenols, folate, and vitamins C and E. Because tomato polyphenols and lycopene possess antioxidant, anti-inflammatory, and cholesterol-lowering properties, these compounds may decrease the risk of cancer and cardiovascular disease.

Cooking and consuming tomatoes with fat, particularly with olive oil, greatly increases the bioavailability of lycopene and polyphenols [Martinez-Huelamo, 2016]. We are often conditioned to think that the cooking process destroys nutrients, but in the case of tomatoes, the reverse is true: Cooking tomatoes in olive oil actually makes them healthier.

A big reason we find tomatoes delicious is the presence of glutamate, an amino acid responsible for the umami flavor in food. Glutamate is a potential migraine trigger, which is why foods or ingredients rich in glutamine can provoke migraine attacks.

In traditional French cooking, the jelly and seeds of the tomato (the pulp) are typically discarded and only the fleshy walls are used. The chef and owner of The Fat Duck in London, Heston Blumenthal, found that the tomato pulp had a very intense umami taste. He asked Professor Donald Mottram and his team at the University of Reading to test the pulp and flesh of the tomato. They confirmed his discovery: The pulp contained four to six times more glutamate than the flesh [Oruna-Concha, 2007]. They also found differences in glutamate levels in different tomato varieties: cherry tomatoes had the highest concentrations of glutamate, while beefsteak tomatoes had the lowest. Glutamate concentrations also rise with tomato ripeness.

To take advantage of the health benefits of tomatoes while lowering the potential for triggering migraine, avoid overly ripe tomatoes and consider removing the pulp before cooking.

KITCHEN TOOLS

 Investing in your kitchen is always a good idea, and you will reap the benefits of less stress and more ease in cooking. With old pans or dull knives it's easy to feel frustration with cooking. Since my goal is to inspire you to want to cook more at home, I've got a few tips that may help. Following are suggestions for what kitchen tools to have on hand to cook not just these recipes, but any meal.

AIR FRYER Air fryers are countertop convection ovens that simulate deep frying without employing a large quantity of oil. It's a great way to crisp up frozen food or lighten up deep-fried recipes. Air fryers come in a variety of sizes and all cook very differently, so it's important to research which one is the best for your family based on what you cook and how many people you typically serve. If you have an Instant Pot and only cook for two to three people, consider an Instant Pot air fryer lid, an attachment for the appliance; it's very convenient and doesn't take up as much space a full-sized air fryer. With my Instant Pot air fryer lid, I cook a fillet of salmon, simply seasoned with salt, pepper, and olive oil, for just 9 to 10 minutes. I microwave some grains and broccoli and have a full meal in 10 minutes. Air-frying can be a healthy alternative to deep-frying, like for my Easy Air-Fried Falafels (page 130), which would normally be deep-fried. An air fryer is also wonderful to reheat quick frozen breakfasts, like hash browns.

You can also use it to dehydrate fruit—a great snack.

CARBON STEEL OR CAST-IRON SKILLET This is a great piece to have for the Roasted Olive Chicken with Couscous (page 187) or anytime you want to get a golden-brown sear on meat or fish, then transfer it to finish cooking in the oven. My favorite brands are MadeIn or Le Creuset, but Lodge also has good, affordable options. Quality pans will make quick work of searing, elevating the flavor, which makes cooking with migraine a little bit easier.

CHEF'S KNIFE If you splurge on one knife, let it be a good chef's knife or santoku knife for everyday chopping. I believe in the value of a good knife so much that I personally had one custom made to fit my hand! It's great to invest in the knife you will use most often, and, properly cared for, it should last a lifetime. A sharp blade will not only make cooking more efficient, but will also keep juice inside the meat, rather than squishing it out all over the cutting board when slicing. Wusthof is very popular among experienced home cooks. It's best to go into a well-stocked kitchenware store and hold a few knives to see what feels best. If you're comfortable with your knife, it will also help prevent any accidents on those bad attack days.

DUTCH OVEN A Dutch oven is a heavy-bottomed, often enameled cast-iron, pot that comes with a tight-fitting lid. It's best used for braises, soups, stews, short ribs, and even to bake homemade bread. It's also deep enough for frying so you won't get splattered, and it maintains the cooking temperature beautifully. Le Creuset and Staub are some of the most popular brands, and they're a worthy investment, but Lodge makes a very affordable one as well. Sometimes you can find a great deal in discount stores. I recommend at least a 6-quart Dutch oven if you cook for 4 people, and a 9-quart pot if you intend to cook for more people or cook very large roasts. I received my first Le Creuset as a gift from my mom when I moved into my own place. Almost 16 years later, it cooks just as well as the first day I got it.

FISH SPATULA Hey, if you're planning on eating all these omega-3s, we need to get you cooking fish properly. And there's nothing worse than trying to flip a fish fillet and having it fall apart. A fish spatula is a large and wide spatula that narrows at the handle. It's not just great for fish! You could use it for pancakes, the Ricotta Kale Fritters (page 68), or omelets. It's large and easy to slide under whatever you're cooking, making you regret ever using the flimsy black one that came in the value pack of kitchen utensils.

HIGH-SPEED BLENDER If you struggle with nausea, as many people with migraine do, smoothies are a great way to get in some nutrition during bad attacks. My Famous Migraine-Fighting Smoothie (page 76) is a go-to for many of my readers. When you're feeling ill, the last thing you want to deal with is a clunky old blender that doesn't blend ice well, leaving little chunks behind. By investing in a good blender, with lots of power and speed, you'll be able to enjoy creamy soups (without adding cream!), homemade sorbets, and sauces, in addition to smoothies. I recommend Ninja, Breville, or Vitamix.

IMMERSION BLENDER You might be asking, "Alicia, do you sell blenders in your spare time?" Hear me out... you need both types. An immersion blender is a stick blender that you insert into mixtures instead of pouring a mixture into a blender container. It's great for homemade mayonnaise, dressings, and soups. It makes blending my Hearty Lentil Soup (page 129) so much easier because you don't have to move a heavy pot over a blender, you can just blend it right in the soup pot, which means one less dish to wash and no accidents! While it may seem pointless if you have a good blender, immersion blenders are inexpensive and can prevent any spills or burns during high pain or dizzy days, which is always a good thing.

INSTANT POT An Instant Pot is basically an electric pressure cooker. Many models have options for other uses, such as making homemade yogurt, cooking rice, simmering soup, and steaming. For me, the main purpose of an Instant Pot is to get food on the table quickly, as it massively cuts down the cooking time. For example, broths that would take 4 to 6 hours to simmer on the stove top cook in just 30 minutes in the Instant Pot. A simple vegetable soup that normally takes 30 to 40 minutes can be made in less than 10 minutes. Rice and mashed potatoes can be ready in 10 minutes. And so on. For meat, I find the short cooking time can take away some of the great flavor you can get from low and slow cooking, so I like to use the Instant Pot when meat isn't the only star of the meal, for example, when folded into tacos, stuffed in pita, or on a salad.

SLOW COOKER A slow cooker doesn't have the pressure-cooking capability but is meant for low and slow cooking. With this method, chicken, beef, or pork can be set to cook at the beginning of the day, and is ready by the time you get home from work. What I love about the slow cooker is it produces good, tender meat. Although an Instant Pot will take you 20 minutes (versus 2 to 8 hours) to cook the same thing, it doesn't have the same depth of flavor that a slow cooker will produce. A slow cooker is a wonderful tool for my Braised Beef (page 217), pulled pork, shredded chicken, and soups. Note: Though many Instant Pots have a slow cooker function, I don't recommend it to replace a slow cooker. I find it doesn't cook as well, and dishes actually take longer to cook than in a slow cooker.

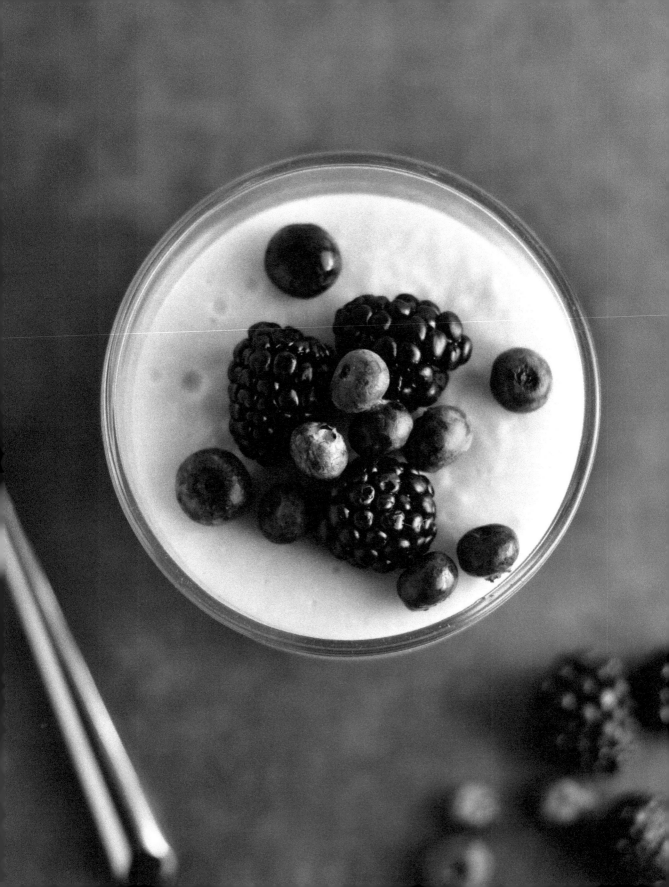

FRUITS

For more recipes featuring fruits, see the index.

THE BENEFITS OF FRUIT

Fruits often feature as a dessert in Mediterranean cuisine. The natural sweetness and sugars are balanced by fruit's fiber content, resulting in a slower blood glucose rise when compared to eating cakes, cookies, or desserts made from refined carbohydrates. Fruits are also rich in antioxidants, which help control inflammatory processes involved in migraine.

BERRIES, like raspberries, blackberries, and blueberries, are superfoods packed with antioxidants, and anti-inflammatory phytochemicals. Strawberries are technically not berries, and although not considered superfoods, are a good source of fiber and antioxidants.

POMEGRANATES originated from the Mediterranean region, and are botanically classified as berries. Pomegranates contain high levels of polyphenols, vitamin C, folate, and fiber, all great nutrients for those with migraine.

APRICOTS are a rich source of fiber, vitamin E, vitamin C, vitamin A, and antioxidants like beta-carotene and polyphenols.

APPLES AND PEARS are highly versatile and can be used in many dishes. They are a moderate source of fiber but do not contain many other nutrients.

WATERMELONS are sweet and juicy, and contain lycopene and moderate amounts of vitamin C, but not many other nutrients. CANTALOUPES contain more antioxidants (e.g., beta-carotene, lutein, zeaxanthin) and vitamin C, compared to watermelons.

The two cultivated forms of CHERRIES are sweet cherries and tart (sour) cherries. Sweet cherries provide a moderate amount of vitamin C, but not many other nutrients. Tart cherries, on the other hand, are rich in vitamin C, vitamin A, and beta-carotene. In addition, tart cherries contain melatonin, which can help with sleep and migraine control.

Sulfites are often used to preserve dried fruit, and give them a more vibrant color. Sulfites are a possible trigger for migraine, so you should limit the use of dried fruit or select dried fruit that does not list sulfur dioxide as a preservative.

COOKING WITH FRUIT

Fruit is incredibly versatile in cooking. Adding berries to salads can provide a hint of sweetness. Berries are also lovely paired with something savory, like cheese or fresh herbs. Of course, berries are wonderful as a dessert when the sweetness is provided directly from the fruit rather than added sugar. Extend the life of fresh berries by giving them a quick vinegar-and-water bath when you bring them home. Fill a large bowl with 3 cups water and 1 cup distilled white vinegar. Add the berries to the solution to eliminate any mold or bacteria growth. Drain and rinse thoroughly, then allow them to dry on a towel. I store mine in small containers lined with paper towels. Make sure they have ventilation and aren't covered with a tight lid, so condensation can evaporate rather than encouraging mold growth.

Tart cherries add a sweet and sour experience to any dish, which is why I love using them as a marinade or in salad dressings. The juice is a wonderful substitute for those sensitive to citrus fruits. Since cherries are naturally rich in melatonin and tryptophan, cherry juice makes a perfect nightcap mocktail to aid in a great night of sleep.

Pomegranate juice and seeds have a tart flavor profile similar to cherries, and the arils or seeds have a delightful burst of flavor that pops in your mouth when you eat them. These are also wonderful on salads, as a salsa for seafood, or mixed in with breakfast puddings.

Melons, apples, and pears can make a wonderful fruit salad and also have different flavors and textures depending on types. My favorite apples to use in cooking are honeycrisp, which taste just like their name. I highly recommend dried apples for high-nausea days. With dried fruits, look for sulfite-free brands, which are generally dull in color. Just like wine, sulfites must be disclosed in the ingredients, most commonly as "sulfur dioxide." Many brands add sulfites to dried apricots because they're an ugly brown color without them. I find a great deal on sulfite-free dried fruit at Trader Joe's.

If you have access to a farmer's market, it will always be the best place to buy fruit, since you're usually getting it super fresh and in season. Organic is ideal, but it can stretch your budget. Buying frozen fruit is a great way to get organic fruit for less. For something like salads, fresh fruit is preferred over softer, watery frozen fruit. But if you're making a smoothie, berry pies, or a compote, frozen will work fine!

Pomegranate Berry Smoothie

MAKES 2 SERVINGS

This smoothie is packed with berry flavor, and it's loaded with antioxidants. I like to use either a mixed frozen berry blend, or a mixture of fresh berries I have on hand. White mulberries are the main species found in Italy and Southern Europe, and are the best ones for this recipe. They have a butterscotch flavor to them and add enough sweetness where you shouldn't need added sugar. Although tough to find in regular grocery stores, dried mulberries are widely available online or in health food stores like Sprouts or Whole Foods. I like to add a scoop of cottage cheese for extra protein, especially since yogurt is a migraine trigger for me. Trust me: You can't even taste it!

3 tablespoons dried mulberries
1 cup frozen mixed berries
1 teaspoon flaxseed meal
1½ tablespoons cottage cheese
¼ cup milk (hemp or oat recommended)
¼ cup pomegranate juice
About ½ cup ice cubes

In a high-speed blender, combine all the berries. Add the flaxseed, cottage cheese, milk, and pomegranate juice. Start blending on low speed, increasing the speed to high as the larger chunks break down and become smooth. If your blender has a tamper, this can help the blending process and should be a first resort over adding more liquid, which can water down the intense berry flavor. Once smooth, add the ice cubes and blend until the ice is fully incorporated and the mixture is smooth.

Divide the smoothie among 2 glasses and serve immediately.

NOTE: For a dairy-free/plant-based option, omit the cottage cheese and use your favorite milk substitute. To boost the protein content you're missing from eliminating the cottage cheese, you can add 1 tablespoon of hemp or chia seeds with the berries, or use hemp milk in place of dairy milk.

TIPS: Flaxseed meal is just ground flaxseed. Buying flaxseed meal saves you the effort of grinding whole flaxseeds yourself! Many recipes in this book use tart cherry juice. If you have some leftover, you can use it instead of the pomegranate juice in this recipe. Occasionally I add ¼ cup frozen spinach to the mix for some extra greens!

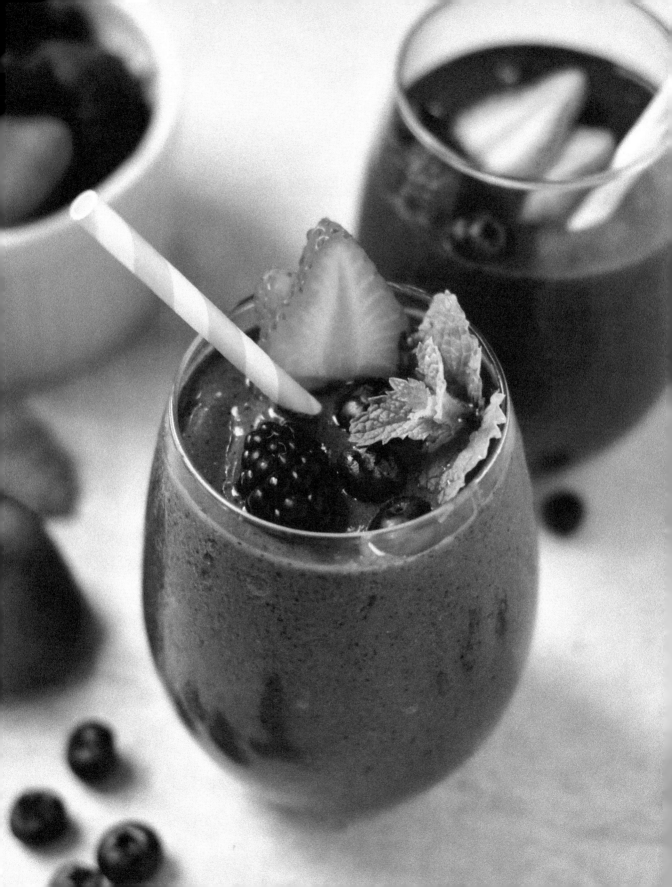

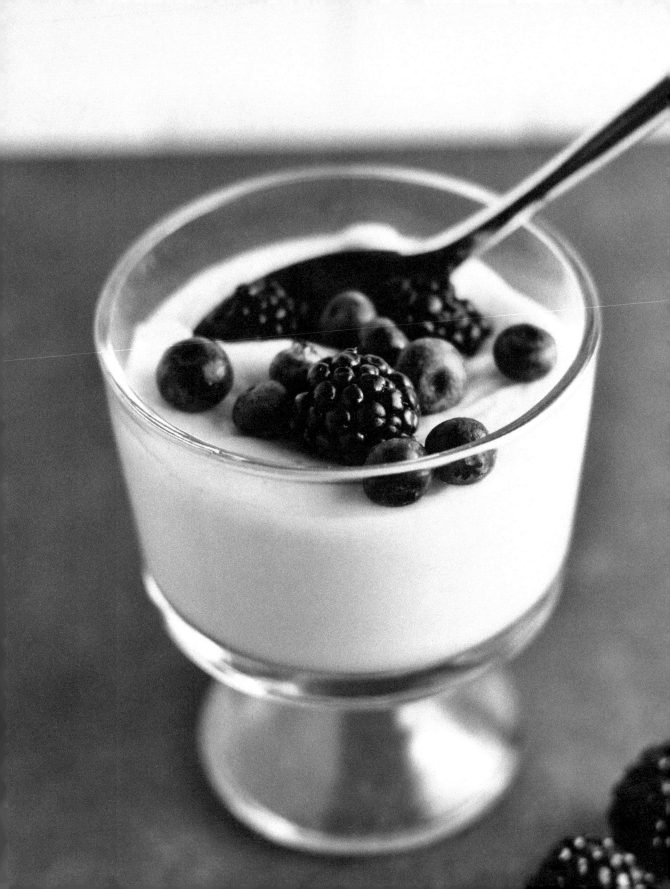

Vanilla-Honey Pudding with Fresh Berries

MAKES 4 INDIVIDUAL PUDDINGS

Sometimes when you have a migraine attack, the only thing that sounds good is something sweet. This light dessert is perfect to keep in the fridge for those moments—or for a sweet, comforting treat anytime.

1½ cups whole milk or oat milk
2 tablespoons cornstarch
2 tablespoons honey
1 teaspoon pure vanilla extract
Pinch of sea salt
1 cup mixed berries

In a saucepan, combine about ⅓ cup of the milk with the cornstarch and whisk until no clumps remain (I find that starting with a smaller amount of milk helps ensure the pudding is totally smooth). Whisk in the rest of the milk, the honey, vanilla, and salt. Set the pan over medium-high heat and cook, whisking consistently, until it reaches a simmer. Continue simmering and whisking until the mixture becomes thick and creamy, 6 to 7 minutes total—the longer you simmer, the thicker the pudding will get. Divide the mixture among 4 serving bowls or cups and place a piece of plastic wrap directly on top of each portion of pudding (this prevents a skin from forming). Refrigerate until cool, at least 2 hours. Store up to 3 or 4 days in the refrigerator.

To serve, remove the plastic wrap and top with fresh mixed berries.

Berry, Beet & Goat Cheese Salad

MAKES 4 SIDE-DISH SERVINGS

Fresh salads abound all over the Mediterranean region, and beets are a popular addition in Turkey. This gorgeous dish is one of my favorites to serve for a date night at home or a holiday meal. My preference is for pre-packed roasted beets over canned. Often you can find these refrigerated in the fresh fruit and vegetable section of the grocery store. Look for a Dijon mustard without white wine/sulfites, like Annie's Organic brand. If you're lucky, a combination of pre-packaged spinach and arugula mix can be found.

DRESSING

1 tablespoon sulfite-free Dijon mustard

1 tablespoon distilled white vinegar

½ tablespoon honey

¼ cup extra virgin olive oil

Kosher salt and black pepper to taste

SALAD

4 ounces fresh arugula

4 ounces fresh spinach

3 to 4 large roasted beets

7 fresh strawberries

⅓ cup blueberries

2 ounces fresh goat cheese, crumbled

In a small bowl, whisk together the Dijon mustard, vinegar, honey, and olive oil until smooth and light yellow in color. Season to taste.

Slice strawberries and beets into bite-size pieces. In a large bowl, mix together spinach and arugula. Portion the spinach and arugula mixture out onto small plates and top each with beets, strawberries, and blueberries evenly. Spoon dressing over the top of each plate, serving any extra on the side, and finish with fresh, crumbled goat cheese.

NOTE: For a dairy-free option, omit the goat cheese.

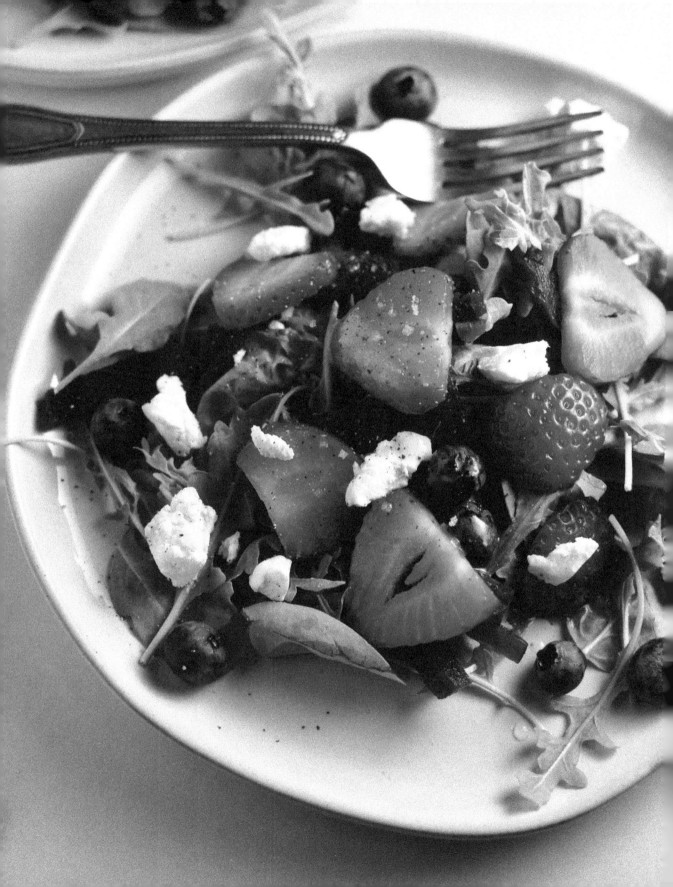

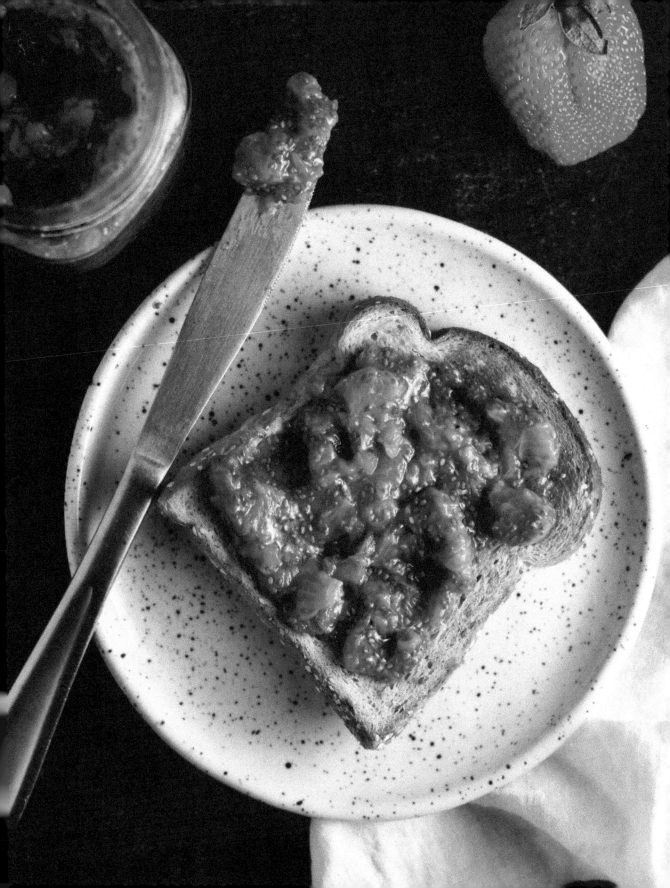

Strawberry-Fennel-Chia Jam

MAKES ABOUT 1 CUP

Normally, making jam at home is a tedious process, but not with this recipe. It's quick and provides a nice boost of omega-3s and antioxidants while also being relatively low in sugar. You can use any fruit, from blueberries and blackberries to cherries! Just use the same amounts as you would the strawberries. Strawberry pairs well with fennel and ginger, but for other fruits, I leave out those additions.

1 pound strawberries, stems removed
⅛ teaspoon fennel seeds
½ teaspoon grated fresh ginger
2 tablespoons chia seeds
2 tablespoons honey

In a small saucepan, heat the strawberries over medium high, stirring occasionally, until the juices release and begin to bubble. Use a potato masher to mash the fruit until your desired consistency is reached (I like a few chunks in there). Stir in the fennel seeds and ginger and allow it to bubble about 1 more minute, then stir in the chia seeds and honey.

Remove the pan from the heat and let cool for about 7 minutes. The jam will thicken as it cools. Stir and transfer to a clean Mason jar. Store in the refrigerator and use within 5 to 7 days.

Melon & Basil Salad

MAKES 6 TO 8 SIDE-DISH SERVINGS

This is one of my favorite summer salads. I love the combination of sweet and savory with the melon and salt, olive oil, and fresh basil. It's a refreshing choice alongside a meal of grilled meat, zucchini, and peppers. Both pomegranate juice and lime juice work well in this recipe, depending on personal preference. If you are sensitive to citrus, leave out the lime zest and juice, and replace with a pinch of sumac, which is just enough to complement the melon.

½ cantaloupe
½ small watermelon
½ honeydew
3 tablespoons chopped fresh basil

DRESSING
2 tablespoons olive oil
1 teaspoon sulfite-free Dijon mustard
1 tablespoon lime juice or pomegranate juice
¼ teaspoon kosher salt
Finely grated zest of 1 lime

Use a small melon baller or chop cantaloupe, watermelon, and honeydew into bite-size pieces (you'll want 2 to 2½ cups of each type). Toss together with fresh basil in a large bowl. Whisk olive oil, Dijon mustard, lime juice or pomegranate juice, kosher salt, and lime zest, if using, until smooth. Pour dressing over the melon salad and toss until all pieces are coated. Serve immediately or chill for up to 1 day.

TIP: Purchase melons that are roughly about the same size so you get equal amounts of each.

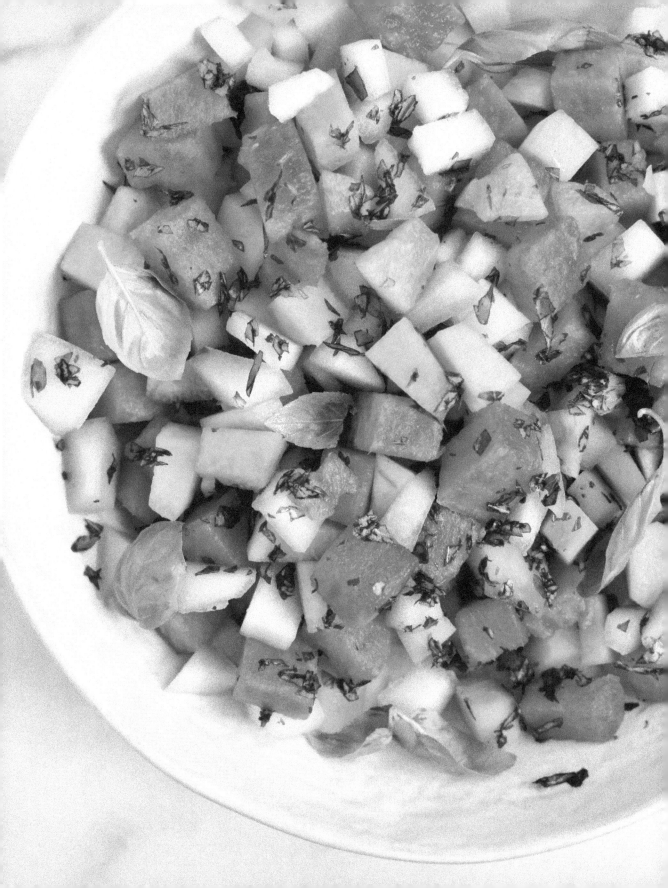

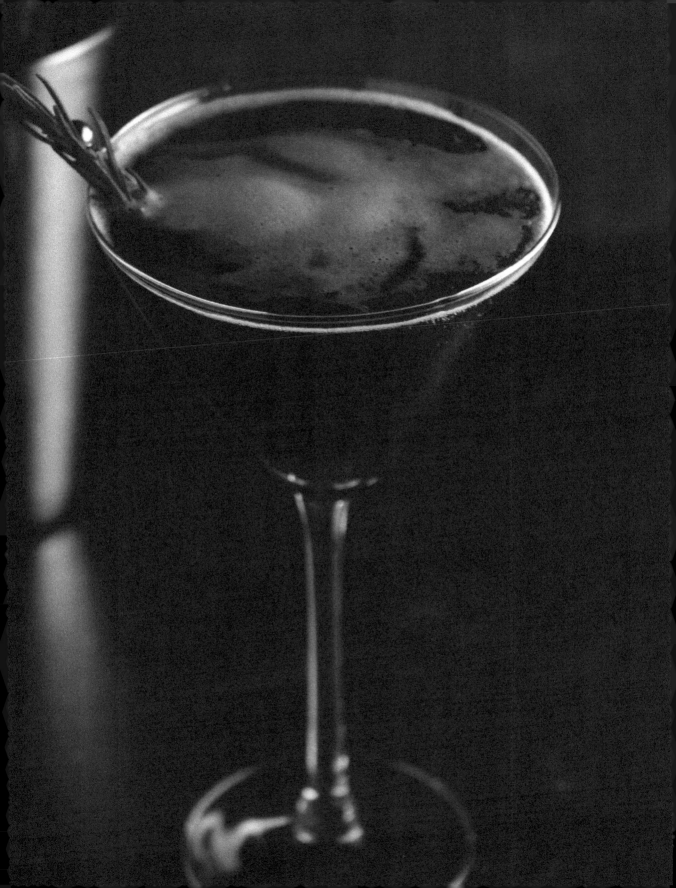

Tart Cherry Nightcap

MAKES 2 SERVINGS

This is the perfect drink to send you off to sweet dreams! This mix of tart cherry juice, chamomile, sparkling water, and a touch of ginger offers melatonin and anti-inflammatory properties to calm the brain and promote a restful night of sleep. Chamomile was once believed to be sacred by the Egyptians and is also valued in Greece for its medicinal qualities. There, it is traditionally used to soothe stomachaches and calm the nervous system.

1 cup tart cherry juice
½ cup brewed chamomile tea
¼ cup apple juice or apple cider
½-inch chunk fresh ginger
Ice
1 bottle (12 ounces) sparkling water or club soda
Small fresh rosemary sprig or thin ginger slice for garnish

In a small saucepan, combine the cherry juice, tea, apple juice, and ginger. Bring to a boil over medium-high heat, then reduce the heat to a low simmer for 5 minutes.

Remove the ginger and allow the mixture to cool.

When ready to serve, put the mixture in a cocktail shaker with ice and shake. Strain the mixture into 2 martini glasses, dividing evenly, and top with a splash of soda. Place a rosemary sprig or slice of ginger in the glass as a garnish and serve right away.

The Best Tart Cherry Marinade

MARINATES UP TO 3 POUNDS OF MEAT OR SHRIMP

This super-easy marinade is my go-to for all things grilled, but I think it pairs best with steak. Use affordable options like flank steak or skirt steak for the best flavor combination. You can find tart cherry juice at most grocery stores, but pomegranate juice will work in a pinch—it, too, provides many health benefits. The combination of garlic and rosemary always reminds me of my trip to Italy where I got to cook with a grandmother named Lucia, who started her own cooking school. She showed me how to use simple herbs to infuse recipes with the best flavors!

1 cup tart cherry juice

3 cloves garlic, minced

1 tablespoon fresh rosemary, chopped

¾ teaspoon kosher salt

In a dish large enough to hold what you plan to marinate, combine the tart cherry juice, minced garlic, fresh rosemary, and kosher salt.

For steak and chicken, marinate covered, in the refrigerator, for 6 to 12 hours for the best flavor, but if you're in a hurry, you can give the meat a light flavor in about 30 minutes. Drain the meat from the marinade, pat dry, and cook to your liking, or see Tart Cherry Grilled Steak on page 214.

For shrimp, marinate covered, in the refrigerator, for 30 minutes to 2 hours, depending on how intense you want the flavor to be. Drain the shrimp from the marinade and cook to according to your preference.

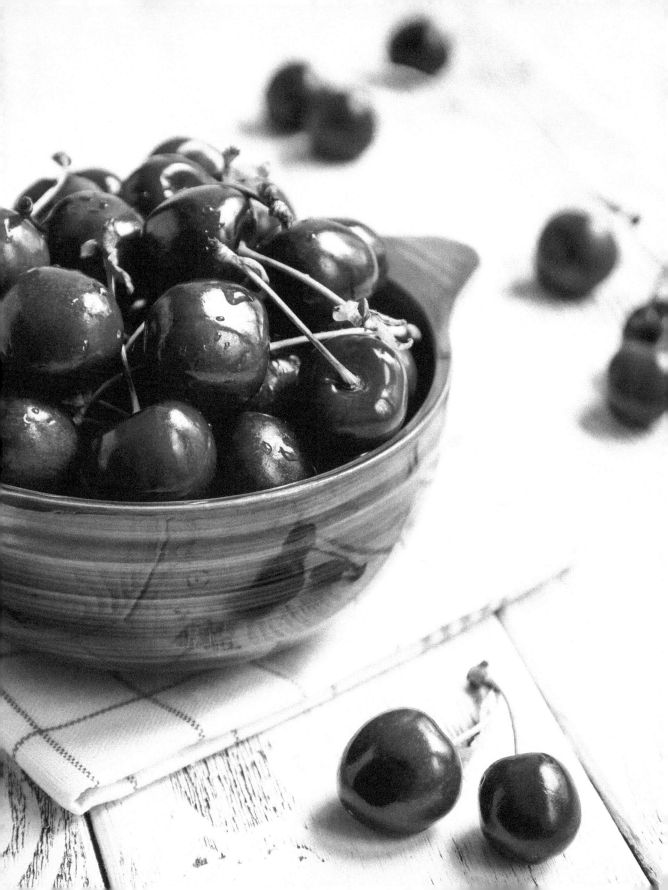

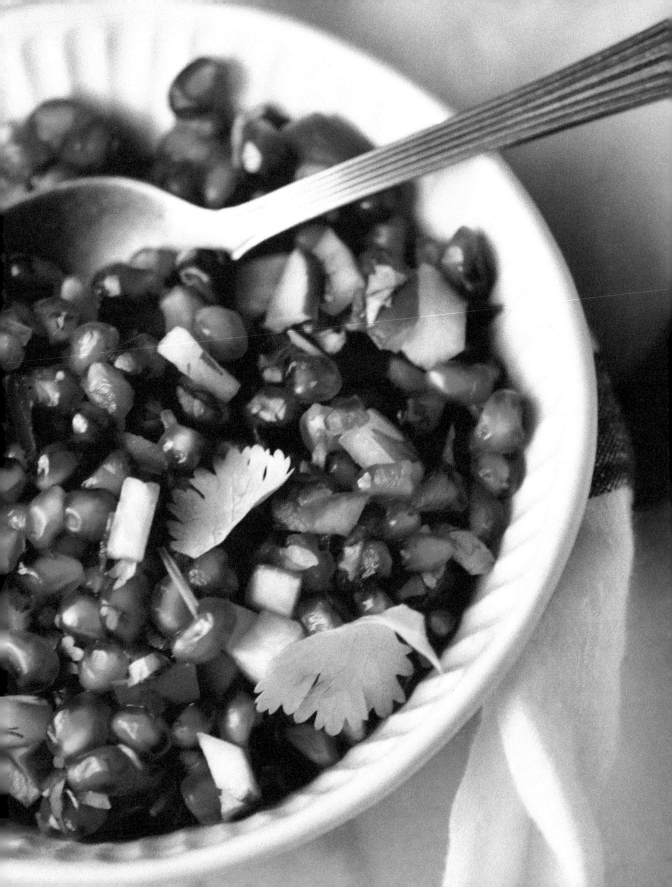

Pomegranate Salsa

MAKES 1 CUP

This pomegranate salsa is amazing on top of grilled seafood or with pita chips as a refreshing and tangy dip. This recipe is wonderful for people who find tomatoes to be a migraine trigger and can't enjoy traditional salsa recipes. Pomegranate arils can be found in the refrigerated fruit section of the grocery store, typically in small cups. This salsa would also be divine on crostini spread with cream cheese or goat cheese for a holiday appetizer.

16 ounces pomegranate arils (seeds)

½ cup chopped red radishes

⅓ cup chopped fresh cilantro

2 teaspoons finely chopped shallots

2 tablespoons green bell pepper, finely chopped (optional)

Juice of ½ lime

In a bowl, mix together the pomegranate seeds, radishes, cilantro, shallots, and green bell pepper, if using. Add the lime juice and stir well. Chill for 30 minutes to allow the flavors to blend.

TIP: If you don't tolerate lime juice well, omit it or substitute 1 teaspoon distilled white vinegar.

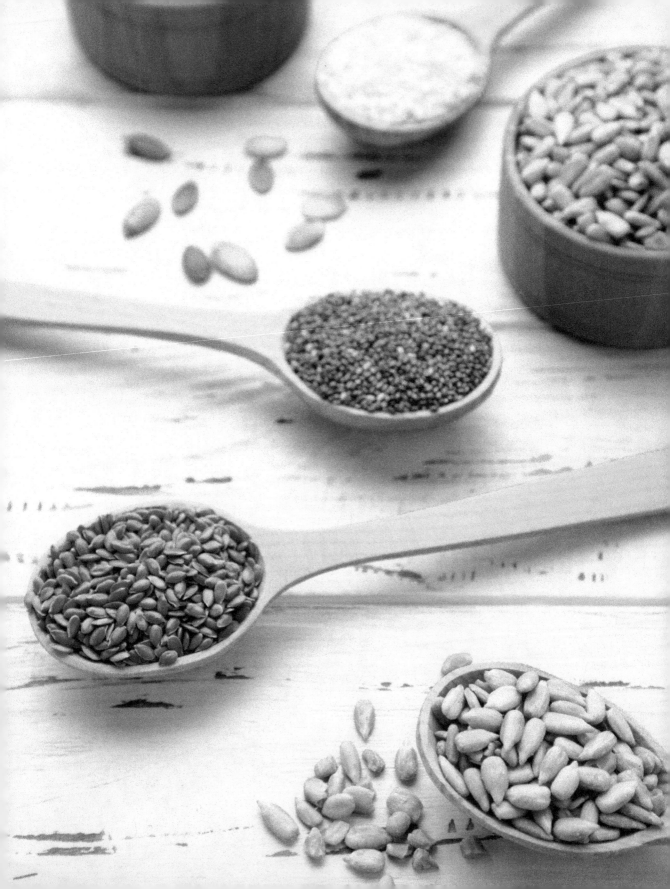

SEEDS

For more recipes featuring seeds, see the index.

THE BENEFITS OF SEEDS

Seeds are nutrient-packed superfoods that should be part of your diet. Sesame seeds are important in Mediterranean cuisine and are rich in a polyphenol called sesamin. Sesame is a component of many Mediterranean spice mixtures and staple ingredients, for example, za'atar and tahini. Pumpkin and sunflower seeds are great sources of fiber, monounsaturated fats, and vitamin E. Flax and chia seeds are rich in omega-3 fatty acids, polyphenols, and fiber. While chia seeds aren't traditionally Mediterranean, they are nutritional powerhouses and fit in very well with this style of eating.

TOASTING SESAME SEEDS

Toasting sesame seeds is a great way to enhance their nutty flavor. To do this, pour the sesame seeds into a small, dry skillet (no oil needed). Place over low heat, stirring often with a wooden spatula, until the seeds are just golden brown and smell nutty, 3 to 4 minutes total. Pour the toasted seeds onto a plate to stop the cooking.

COOKING WITH SEEDS

Using nuts and seeds in cooking is a wonderful way to add protein and healthy fat to any meal, and they make a filling snack. However, I found out through an elimination diet that nuts are one of my big migraine triggers. As such, the recipes in this chapter all feature seeds, which I find are really under-used in recipes when compared with nuts. I hope you'll find them to be just as enjoyable, but if you're a big nut fan, feel free to substitute your favorite nuts or nut butters in these recipes.

SESAME SEEDS are a popular ingredient in Mediterranean countries. I use them as a topping for salads, in my Easy Air-Fried Falafels (page 130), and in energy balls for snacking. Tahini, which is sesame paste, has an earthy flavor and creamy texture that is wonderful for sauces, dressings, and in smoothies.

SUNFLOWER SEEDS and PUMPKIN SEEDS (also known as pepitas) are the best when lightly roasted, which you can do by toasting them in the oven on a baking sheet or in a dry pan, flipping until lightly browned on both sides. Sometimes you can purchase them pre-roasted and unsalted, but they turn rancid faster than raw seeds. Store raw seeds in the refrigerator or freezer for the longest shelf life. Sunflower seed butter is widely available, and I find roasted and unsweetened to have the best flavor. Pumpkin seed butter is a little harder to find, but available online or at health food stores. You can also make your own with a good quality food processor.

CHIA, FLAX SEEDS, AND HEMP SEEDS are all wonderful ways to add nutrients to smoothies and breakfast recipes. Chia seeds are not native to the Mediterranean, but their high nutrient value is compatible with the principles of the Mediterranean diet. When chia is mixed with liquid, it expands and makes a thick pudding or jam. Hemp seeds and hemp milk are high in protein and make a great plant-based milk substitute. I find the flavor really earthy, so I tend to use them for pestos, in smoothies, or in granola, where the taste is mellowed by the other flavors.

Pumpkin Seed Smoothie

MAKES 2 SERVINGS

The star ingredient of this smoothie is creamy, roasted pumpkin seed butter which you can find online through places like 88 Acres (88acres.com) or in natural foods stores. If you can't locate it, sunflower seed butter works well, or nut butters (I highly recommend almond butter), if they don't trigger your migraine symptoms. Dried white mulberries can also be found through an online source or at health food stores. Here the healthy omega-6-rich pumpkin seeds are balanced with the omega-3s in the flax seeds.

3 tablespoons pumpkin seed butter

¼ cup dried white mulberries

2 teaspoons honey

1 tablespoon flaxseed meal

1 tablespoon Greek yogurt (if tolerated) or cottage cheese

1 cup oat milk (or any milk you like)

1½ to 2 cups ice cubes

In a blender, combine the pumpkin seed butter, mulberries, honey, flax seeds, cottage cheese or yogurt, and oat milk. Blend until everything is smooth and creamy. Add the ice cubes and blend until the ice is fully incorporated and the mixture is smooth.

Divide the smoothie among 2 glasses and serve immediately.

NOTE: For a dairy-free smoothie, replace the yogurt or cottage cheese with 2 tablespoons frozen riced cauliflower, which adds creaminess.

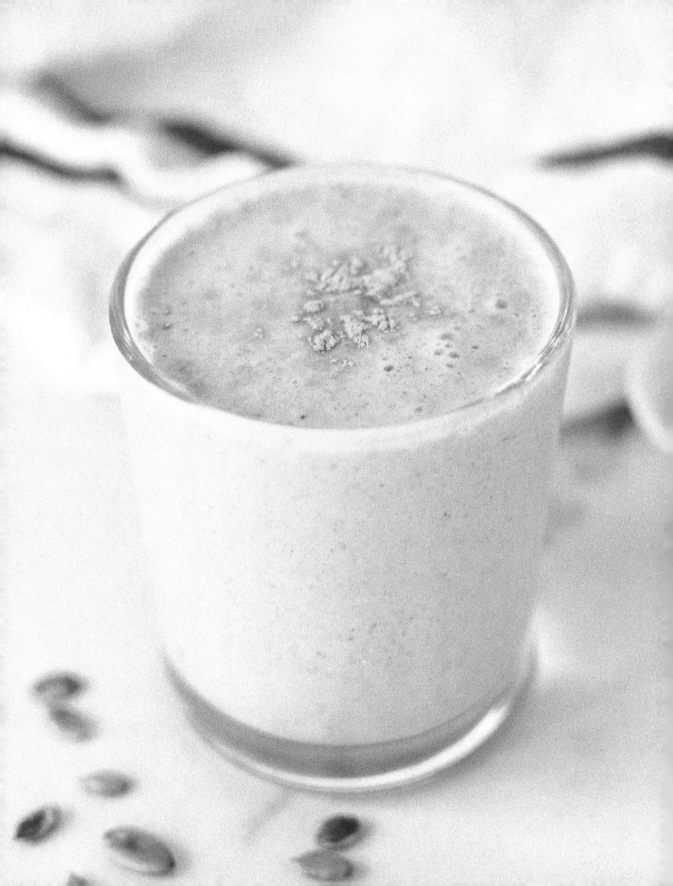

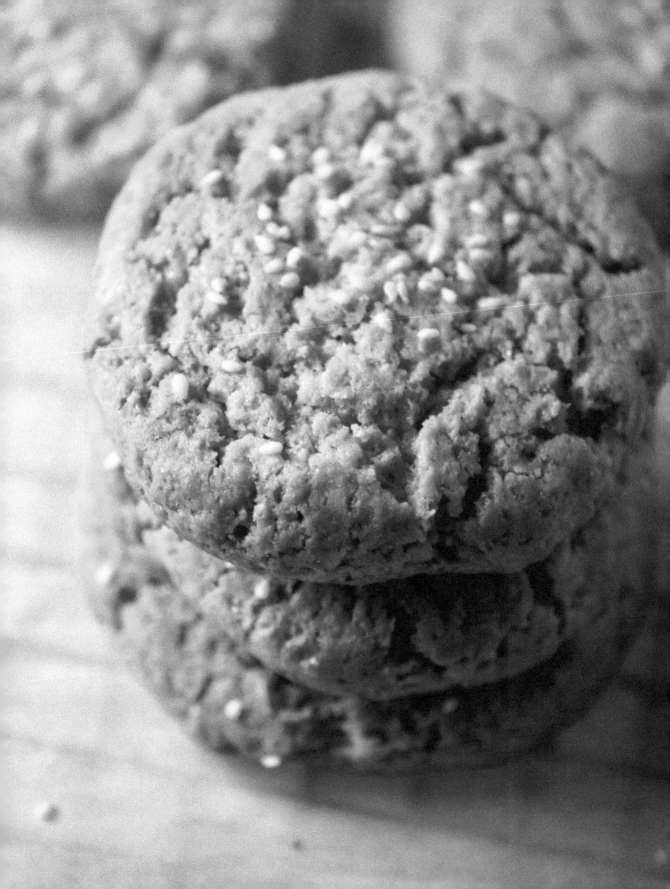

Honey Tahini Cookies

MAKES 18 COOKIES

The flavor of these sesame and honey cookies is distinctly Mediterranean. Unlike crunchy Italian sesame cookies, this recipe makes a softer, almost gooey, cookie. Turn to page 54 for instructions on toasting sesame seeds. Store-bought tahini can have a wide range of flavors, so taste yours before using it for this recipe and make sure it's well mixed with the oil in the package. My favorite tahini brands include Krinos and Trader Joe's.

½ cup tahini
⅓ cup granulated sugar
⅓ cup honey
1 teaspoon pure vanilla extract
1 large egg
1½ cups all-purpose flour
1 teaspoon baking soda
¼ teaspoon kosher salt
About 1 tablespoon toasted sesame seeds for topping

In a large bowl, combine the tahini, sugar, honey, and vanilla, stirring with a rubber spatula until fully incorporated. Add the egg and mix until smooth.

In a small bowl, combine the flour, baking soda, and salt and mix with a spoon. Slowly stir the flour mixture into the tahini mixture, stirring with the rubber spatula to incorporate everything.

Pour the sesame seeds onto a plate. Using your hands, shape the dough into 1½- to 2-inch balls. Roll each ball lightly in the toasted sesame seeds and set aside on a rimmed baking sheet as you work. Chill the dough balls for at least 1 hour to firm up.

Preheat the oven to 350°F and line a large, rimmed baking sheet with parchment paper.

Place the dough balls at least 1 inch apart on the prepared baking sheet. Place on the middle rack in the oven and bake until light golden brown, watching carefully to make sure they don't get too dark, 9 to 11 minutes. These cook FAST, especially on the bottoms. In my oven, 10 minutes is the perfect amount of time.

Remove the cookies from the oven and allow them to cool on the baking sheet for 2 to 3 minutes. Serve warm, or transfer to a wire rack to cool completely and store in an airtight container for up to 5 days... but they never last that long.

NOTE: For gluten-free cookies, use gluten-free 1:1 all-purpose baking flour instead of wheat flour.

Anti-Inflammatory Chia Pudding

MAKES 1 SERVING

This chia pudding is the perfect make-ahead breakfast. It combines pain-fighting ginger and anti-inflammatory turmeric, some of the key ingredients in "golden milk," which gets its name from the golden color turmeric provides. Make a large batch and spoon into individual mason jars for a quick breakfast or snack on the go. Turmeric tends to be a strong flavor, so if you're not used to it, start with ¼ teaspoon and add more as needed. If you're a huge golden milk fan, go for the full amount. Black pepper is needed to boost the anti-inflammatory power of the curcumin in turmeric, so you get the most health benefits from this recipe. Use whatever milk you like best. For a decadent treat, top with whipped cream or coconut cream.

½ cup chia seeds

2 cups milk

1 teaspoon pure vanilla extract

¼ to ½ teaspoon ground turmeric

¼ teaspoon ground cardamom

½ teaspoon ground ginger

Pinch of freshly cracked black pepper

1 tablespoon honey (if using unsweetened milk)

Chopped fresh fruit such as mango for serving, optional

Quick Seed Granola (page 63) for serving, optional

In a bowl, combine the chia seeds, milk, vanilla, turmeric, cardamom, ginger, black pepper, and honey, if using, until thoroughly blended. Refrigerate for 10 minutes.

Remove the mixture from the refrigerator and whisk again, making sure to get to any hidden chia seeds in the corners. Cover the bowl and refrigerate until the pudding has fully set up, about 2 hours or up to overnight. Store in the refrigerator for up to 5 days.

To serve, layer or top with fruit of your choice (I like chopped mangoes) or Quick Seed Granola or just eat it plain!

NOTE: For a dairy-free option, use oat milk.

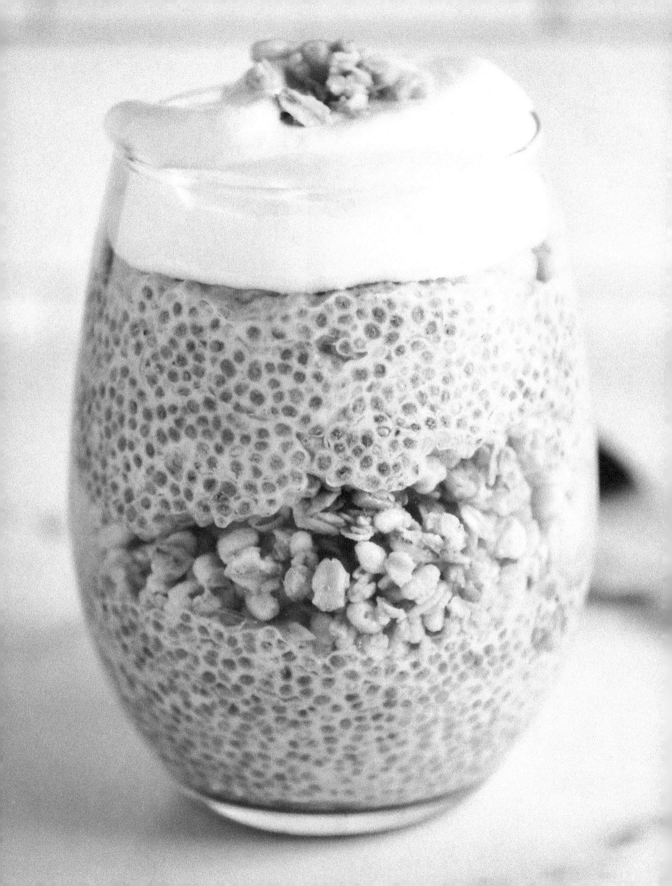

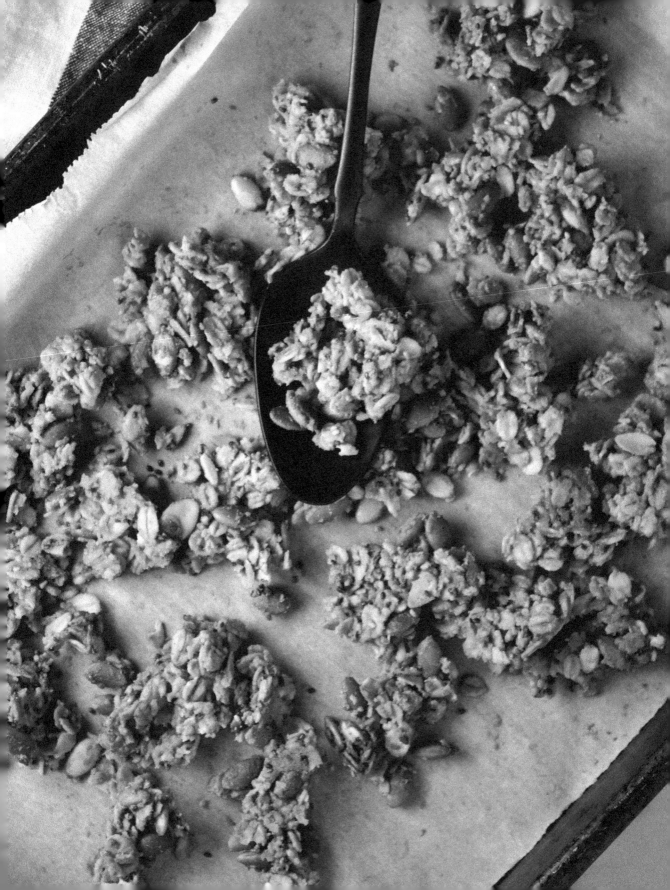

Quick Seed Granola

MAKES ABOUT 3 CUPS

Granola can be super delicious without nuts! This is a softer granola recipe that's great for snacking and, best of all, it cooks super-fast. Start with pre-toasted pumpkin seeds to save time. Use this to top smoothie bowls, ice cream, or Greek yogurt (if tolerated) or cottage cheese and fruit for breakfast. If you're using unsalted sunflower seed butter, add ¼ teaspoon salt to the mixture. If you'd like to use nuts, I recommend switching out the sunflower seed butter for almond or pecan butter, but leaving the pepitas in.

¼ cup unsweetened, salted sunflower seed butter

¼ cup plus 2 teaspoons honey

1½ cups rolled oats

½ cup roasted, unsalted pumpkin seeds (pepitas)

1 tablespoon chia seeds

1 teaspoon pure vanilla extract

¼ teaspoon ground cardamom

Preheat the oven to 325°F. Line a large, rimmed baking sheet with parchment paper.

In a large bowl, combine the sunflower seed butter and honey, mixing with a wooden spoon until blended. Stir in the oats, pumpkin seeds, chia seeds, vanilla extract, and cardamom. Spread the mixture on the parchment paper, spreading it out as much as you can. Bake until golden brown, watching carefully as it can burn easily, 13 to 16 minutes.

Remove the granola from the oven and allow it to cool on the baking sheet for at least 30 minutes. The granola will clump together as it cools; right out of the oven, it will seem too soft.

Serve right away or store in an airtight container for up to 1 week.

TIP: If you're like me and find yourself sensitive to fermented dairy such as yogurt, I highly recommend trying cottage cheese. Hate the texture? Yeah, me too! The best way around this is to blend it in a food processor. Lumpy cottage cheese becomes light, fluffy, and super creamy. It's so delicious this way, drizzled with a bit of honey and, of course, this granola.

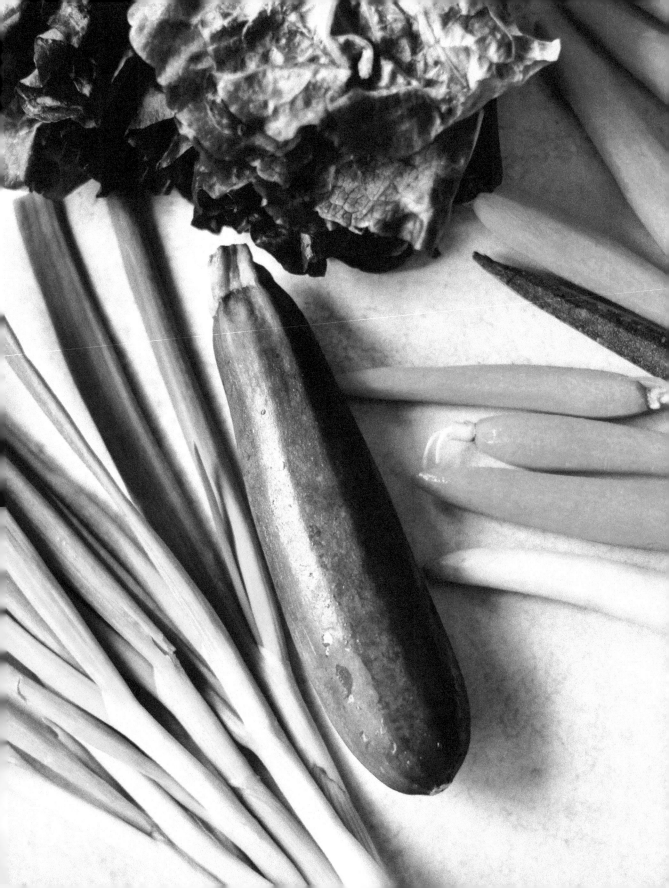

VEGETABLES

For more recipes featuring vegetables, see the index.

THE BENEFITS OF VEGETABLES

In the Mediterranean, vegetables feature prominently. Many vegetables contain nutrients that are not only essential for optimal health but can also help reduce migraine activity.

ARTICHOKES, popular in Italian and Spanish cuisine, are a species of thistle. They're loaded with nutrients, in particular fiber, folate, and vitamin C, and very high in antioxidants.

ASPARAGUS is an amazing source of fiber, folate, vitamin C, vitamin E, and antioxidants.

BEETS have an earthy flavor, and are rich in folate, copper, manganese, and fiber. The bright color of beets is due to betalains, which are powerful antioxidants.

BELL PEPPERS are a low-calorie, low-carb, flavor-packed vegetable that are rich in nutrients and antioxidants. Green peppers are harvested earlier, while red peppers are left on the vine the longest. As such, red peppers have much more beta-carotene and vitamin C.

CARROTS are a nutritious, low-carb, high-fiber root vegetable that add both flavor and crunchiness to food. The bright orange color is due to beta-carotene, a potent antioxidant that is transformed into vitamin A when ingested.

EGGPLANTS (technically considered fruits) are a wonderful low-calorie source of fiber, antioxidants, manganese, vitamin C, and folate. The darker-colored eggplants contain higher levels of antioxidants.

GREEN BEANS are the unripe fruit of the common bean. They not only provide texture and flavor, but are high in fiber and protein, as well as various nutrients like vitamin C, manganese, and folate.

LEAFY GREEN VEGETABLES (e.g., kale, cabbage, broccoli, Brussels sprouts, Swiss chard, spinach, arugula, and more) are great sources of fiber, riboflavin, magnesium, folate, vitamin C, and antioxidants. The humble cabbage has been cultivated for thousands of years and is used in many cuisines. It is rich in vitamins A, B2, B6, and C, as well as folate, iron, fiber, and polyphenols.

MUSHROOMS (e.g., button, cremini, portobello) are a low-calorie and delicious source of vitamin B2, folate, vitamin B6, vitamin C, and antioxidants that can add a whole new flavor dimension to a dish. Mushrooms may contain high levels of glutamate; unsurprisingly, the more intense the flavor of the mushroom, the higher the levels of glutamate. For example, dried shiitake mushrooms have an amazingly rich umami flavor, and, thus, high levels of glutamate. White button mushrooms, which are mildly flavored, have a low glutamate content. Remember, too much glutamate may aggravate migraine activity.

SUMMER SQUASH AND ZUCCHINI are also low-carb, low-calorie vegetables that are high in vitamins A, C, and B6, and magnesium, manganese, folate, fiber, antioxidants, and beta-carotene.

SWEET POTATOES are more nutritious than regular potatoes, with higher levels of vitamin B6, vitamin C, copper, manganese, fiber, and, especially, vitamin A. Despite the name, sweet potatoes have a lower glycemic index compared to potatoes; this means that they affect blood sugar levels to a lesser degree.

COOKING WITH VEGETABLES

The recipes in this chapter are some of my favorites and show how versatile vegetables can be.

In general, when buying most vegetables, you want to look for a smooth, firm, blemish-free surface and choose ones that are heavy for their size. Here are some specific things to look for when buying certain vegetables.

For ARTICHOKES, I recommend canned or frozen, unless you have the time to steam and peel fresh (and if you do, you're amazing). Some of my readers are sensitive to citric acid, so I notice that rinsing canned artichokes in a colander under cool water helps take away some of the tinny flavor and also make them more well tolerated.

For ASPARAGUS, choose brightly colored stalks that are firm. To store, trim about 1 inch from the woody ends and place them in a shallow cup of water in the fridge. This will help them to stay fresh longer.

When choosing BRUSSELS SPROUTS, look for fresh outer leaves without dark or wilted edges. With cauliflower and broccoli, look for tightly packed florets that are creamy white or green and not spotted or yellow.

I often like to buy GREEN BEANS pre-packaged, just to make life a little bit easier. The stringy ends are usually snipped, and the beans are ready to be cooked.

When buying LEAFY GREENS, look for vibrant colors and avoid wilted edges. The leaves should be firm and crisp, not limp or rubbery.

For MUSHROOMS, look for tops that are white or brown, without bruises or blemishes. To clean them, wet a paper towel and rub off the dirt from the cap to stem. Trim the very end of the stem, which is

tough. Rinsing mushrooms under water causes them to absorb more moisture and they will not brown well or have the best flavor.

SWEET POTATOES can come in many varieties, but I recommend Beauregard (which is the most common one sold at stores), Jewel, and Garnet. Sometimes these are also called yams. Avoid purple sweet potatoes, with a white skin and purple inside, or Japanese sweet potatoes, which have a purple exterior. These will be starchier and won't have the same flavor.

To make life a little bit easier on days you don't feel well, use PRE-CUT AND WASHED VEGETABLES.

As for VEGETABLE BROTH, make your own by adding scrap vegetables to an Instant Pot and pouring in 8 to 10 cups of water. Following the manufacturer's directions, cook for 30 minutes and release the pressure. Strain out the vegetables and adjust the seasoning. If you want a quick solution, look for a prepared vegetable broth with simple ingredients and no "natural flavors," which can mimic MSG. Low-sodium brands are my favorite because it's easy to adjust the seasoning to your liking later.

Ricotta Kale Fritters

MAKES 12 FRITTERS

Want to get your family to eat 12 cups of greens in one sitting? Stop laughing and I'll give you a secret—these fritters! It's important to use good ricotta here. A quality brand like Calabro, BelGiosio, or Liuzzi is smooth and creamy, not gritty, which you'll get with brands that add gums. Trust me: It's worth paying an extra dollar for good ricotta! Top with a touch of whipped cottage cheese (or yogurt) and grated lemon zest, if tolerated. These are best served with a simple grilled protein, or on their own as a vegetarian dish. I personally like the mixture of kale and spinach, but you can substitute other greens, if you prefer.

6 cups chopped kale, woody stems removed

6 cups fresh spinach leaves, coarse stems removed

¼ cup water

1 cup all-purpose flour

1 teaspoon kosher salt

1½ teaspoons baking powder

1 teaspoon paprika

½ teaspoon garlic powder

1 cup ricotta cheese

¾ cup milk

2 large eggs

2 to 3 tablespoons olive oil

Whipped cottage cheese, or Greek yogurt, if tolerated, for serving

Finely grated lemon zest, for serving (optional)

Put the kale, spinach, and water in a large skillet. Cover and cook over medium-high heat, stirring occasionally, until the greens are wilted, about 10 minutes. If the water evaporates during cooking, add a splash of water as needed. Transfer the wilted greens to a colander and run under cold running water to stop the cooking. Place the greens in a clean dishtowel or on several layers of paper towels and squeeze out as much moisture as possible. You should have roughly 2 cups of greens.

In a large bowl, combine the flour, salt, baking powder, paprika, and garlic powder. In a small bowl, combine the ricotta, milk, and eggs, whisking until smooth. Pour the ricotta mixture into the flour mixture and add the greens. Stir with a rubber spatula until everything is incorporated.

Add the olive oil to a large nonstick skillet and place over medium heat. To make each fritter, add about 3 tablespoons of the greens mixture to the pan, which should be about 2 to 3 inches in diameter. Add additional fritters to the pan, leaving an inch of space between each one. These don't spread much, but do puff up! Cook the fritters until golden brown on the bottom, about 3 minutes. Flip and cook until the other side is golden brown, another 3 minutes. Transfer the fritters to a paper towel-lined plate and keep warm while you cook the remaining mixture in the same manner.

Serve warm with a dollop of whipped cottage cheese or Greek yogurt and grated lemon zest, if desired.

NOTE: For a gluten-free option, use gluten-free all-purpose flour.

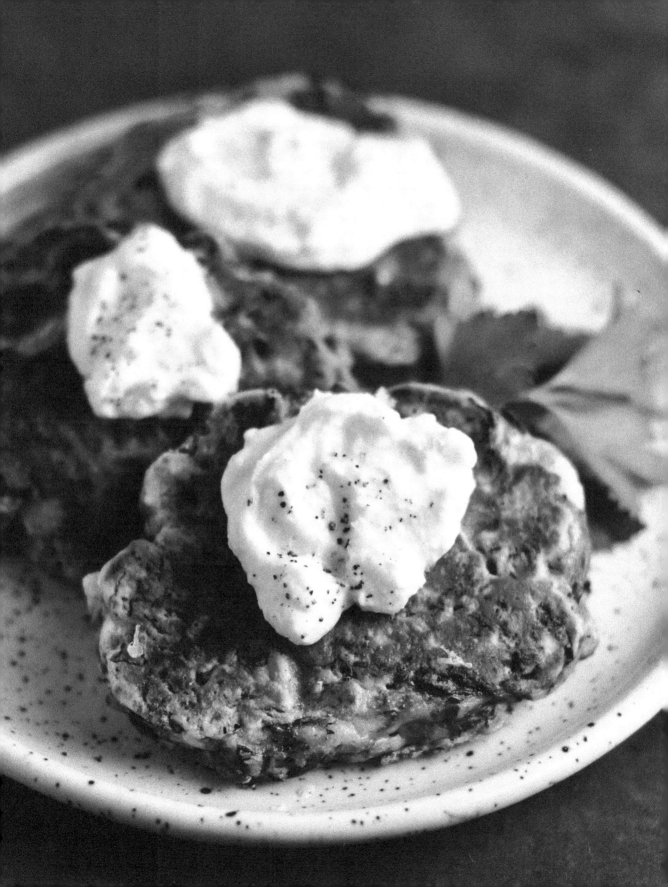

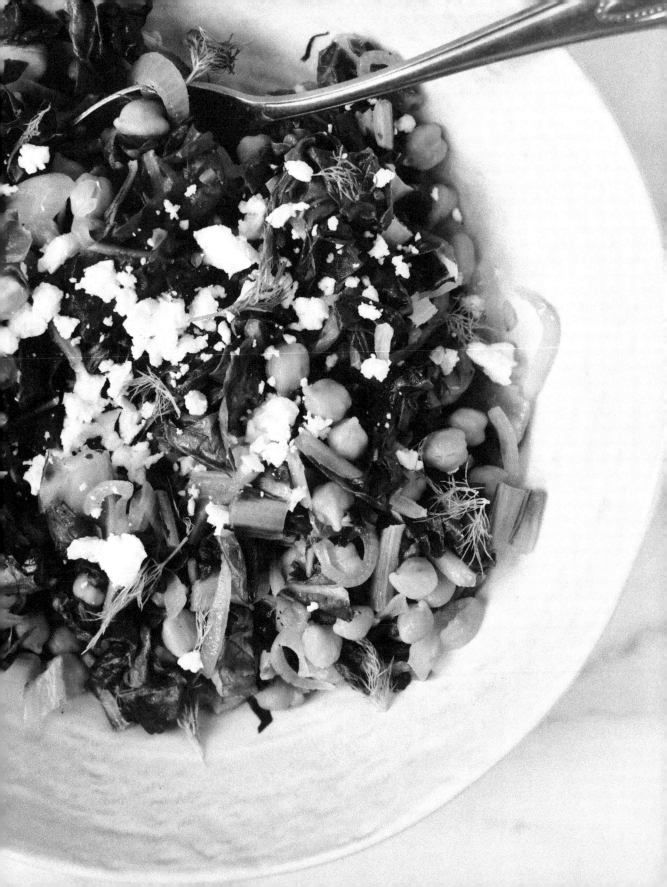

Garbanzo, Shallot & Chard Salad

MAKES 4 TO 6 SIDE-DISH SERVINGS

This nutrient-packed salad combines leafy greens, chickpeas (for extra protein!),
and shallots with fresh dill and feta or halloumi. It's perfect with a fried or poached egg
on top for a healthy breakfast or as a side dish to grilled fish. When choosing feta,
fresh-packed in water is usually the best flavor and texture.

2 large bunches Swiss chard, washed well

1 teaspoon olive oil

1 large shallot, chopped

One 15-ounce can garbanzo beans, rinsed and drained

1 tablespoon fresh lemon juice or distilled white vinegar

2 tablespoons minced fresh dill

¼ cup crumbled feta or cubed halloumi cheese

Kosher salt and freshly ground black pepper

Separate the chard leaves from the stems. Discard the large thick parts of the stem and chop the smaller parts of the stems—these add a great crunch to the salad. Roughly chop the chard leaves into small pieces.

Add the olive oil to a large skillet over medium heat. Add the chopped chard stems, shallots, and garbanzo beans and cook, stirring frequently with a wooden spoon, until the stems and shallots have softened, 3 to 5 minutes. Add the chard leaves and cook until wilted, 1 to 2 minutes.

Transfer the mixture to a serving bowl and top with lemon or vinegar, dill, and feta. Toss to combine and season to taste with kosher salt and pepper. Serve warm or at room temperature.

NOTE: For a dairy-free/plant-based option, omit the cheese.

Sesame Brussels Sprout Salad

MAKES 4 SIDE-DISH SERVINGS

Here, shredded Brussels sprouts are tossed in a creamy honey-tahini dressing for a perfect pairing to any Mediterranean meal. I like to buy pre-shredded Brussels sprouts, which you can find packaged at most grocery stores. Pair this dish with Easy Air-Fried Falafels (page 130) and pita bread for a full meal. Tahini can have a wide range of flavors, so be sure to taste yours before using. For best results, you want a tahini that is mixed with oil and has a drippy texture. My favorite brands include Krinos and Trader Joe's.

¼ cup tahini

2 tablespoons distilled white vinegar

2 tablespoons warm water

1 tablespoon honey

1 teaspoon sesame oil

¼ teaspoon kosher salt

10 ounces shredded Brussels sprouts

Kosher salt and freshly ground black pepper

2 teaspoons toasted sesame seeds

In a large bowl, combine the tahini, vinegar, water, honey, sesame oil, and salt, and whisk until combined. Add shredded Brussels sprouts and toss until well coated. Taste and adjust the seasonings, adding salt and pepper as needed.

Let the dressed Brussels sprouts sit until they begin to soften, and the flavors develop, at least 10 minutes. Sprinkle with the sesame seeds. Serve at room temperature.

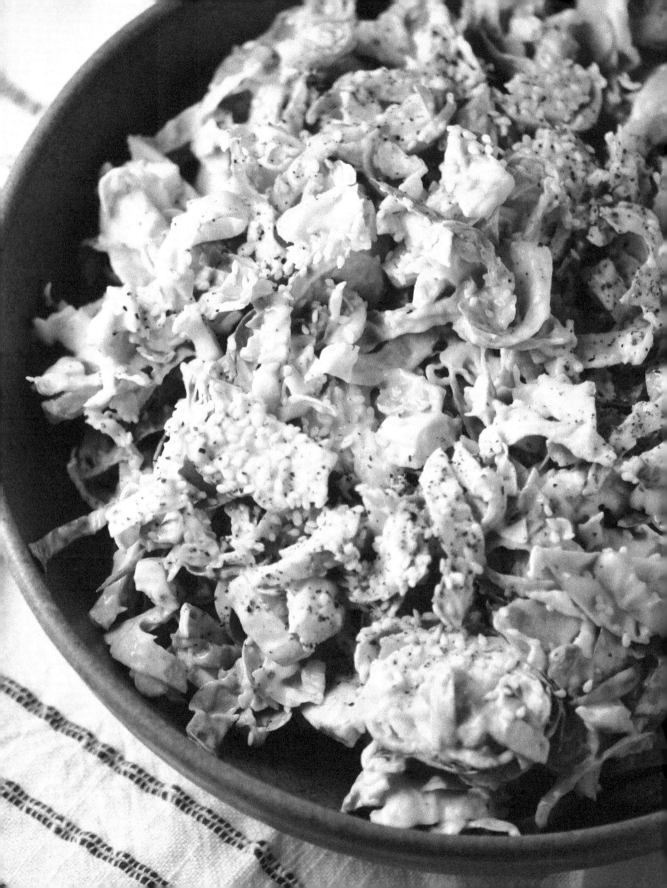

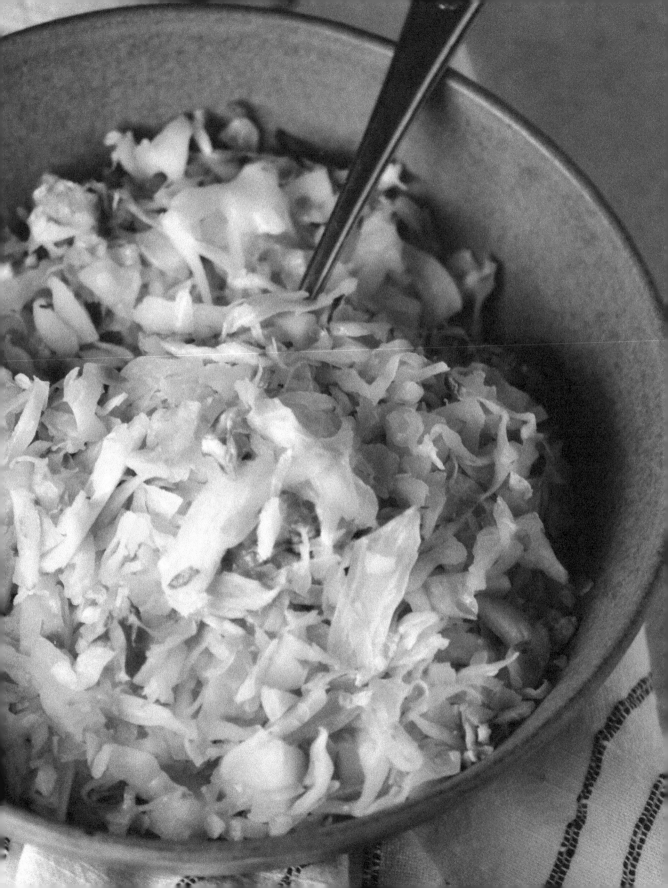

Sautéed Cabbage & Apples

MAKES 4 SIDE-DISH SERVINGS

The quickest way to make this recipe is to buy pre-shredded cabbage. If you're using a whole cabbage, discard any damaged outer leaves, rinse it under cold water, and pat dry. Cut the cabbage in half vertically through the core, then cut those pieces in half. Remove the tough inner core, then run a large chef's knife down the sides of each section, slicing the leaves as thinly as possible. This recipe is wonderful with roast chicken or seared salmon.

2 tablespoons olive oil

1 cup peeled and chopped honeycrisp apple (½-inch pieces)

One 10-ounce package shredded green cabbage

½ teaspoon fresh thyme leaves

½ teaspoon kosher salt

¼ teaspoon freshly ground black pepper

In a large skillet, warm the olive oil over medium heat. Add the apple pieces and sauté briefly to soften, about 30 seconds. Add the cabbage, fresh thyme leaves, salt, and pepper, and let the mixture sit for 2 minutes. Stir with a wooden spoon and continue to cook, stirring occasionally, as the cabbage softens and turns light brown, about 10 minutes total. Taste and adjust the seasonings. Serve warm.

Famous Migraine-Fighting Smoothie

MAKES 2 SERVINGS

This recipe is popular in my circle for helping people on migraine attack days. Easy to whip up, the simple ingredients each help to bring down pain and inflammation, while the light flavors are easy to stomach if nausea is a factor. Drinking the smoothie is also a great way to fit some extra greens into your diet. I like to use oat milk for this recipe, but any type of milk will work. Arugula offers a great peppery flavor that complements the pear well.

¾ cup chopped pear, skin on

2 teaspoons grated fresh ginger

¾ cup fresh spinach or arugula

¾ cup milk

2 teaspoons flaxseed meal

1 cup ice cubes

1 teaspoon honey (optional)

In a blender, combine the pear, ginger, arugula, milk, and seeds and blend until smooth. Add the ice cubes and blend until the ice is fully incorporated and the mixture is smooth and frothy. Taste and add honey, if desired.

Divide the smoothie among 2 glasses and serve immediately.

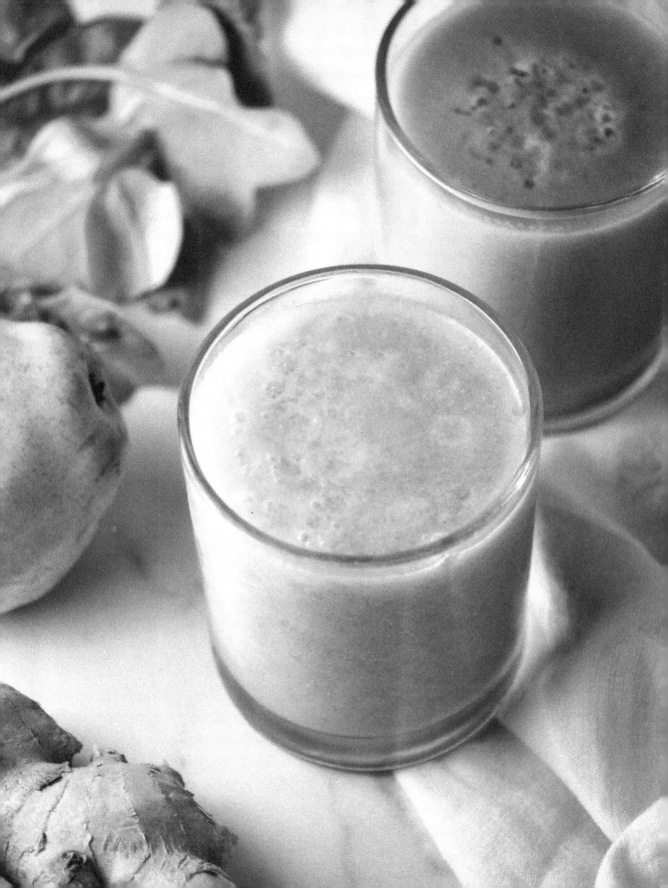

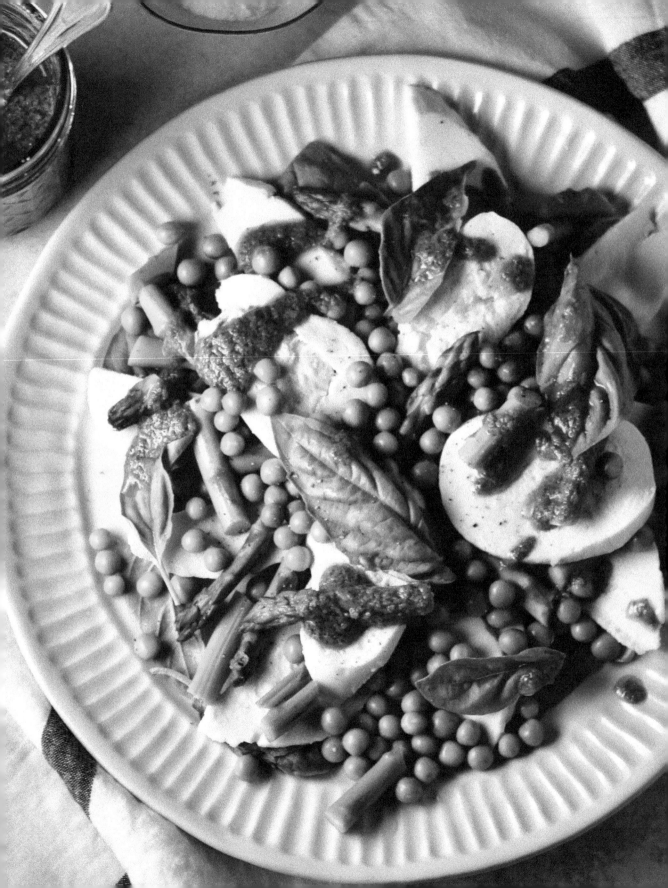

Asparagus & Pea Salad with Basil Vinaigrette

MAKES 4 SIDE-DISH SERVINGS

Here is a perfect spring salad featuring asparagus and peas in their prime season. Par-boiling the vegetables until slightly soft, but still with a nice crispness, makes them the perfect base to pair with creamy mozzarella cheese. The basil vinaigrette is amazing on salads and sandwiches, or even mixed with pasta for a pasta salad. It will keep for up to 1 week in the fridge.

BASIL VINAIGRETTE

2 cups fresh basil leaves

1 small garlic clove

½ cup extra-virgin olive oil

2 tablespoons distilled white vinegar

1 small shallot, chopped (about 2 tablespoons)

¼ teaspoon each kosher salt and freshly ground black pepper

SALAD

10 ounces fresh shelled English peas

10 ounces fresh asparagus, woody ends trimmed, and cut into 2-inch pieces

One 8-ounce ball fresh mozzarella cheese, thinly sliced

10 fresh basil leaves

To make the vinaigrette, in a small food processor, combine the 2 cups basil leaves, the garlic clove, olive oil, vinegar, shallot, salt, and pepper. Pulse a few times to break down the larger pieces, and then blend until smooth. Set aside.

To make the salad, fill a large bowl with water and ice. Bring a saucepan of water to a boil over high heat. Add the shelled peas and asparagus at the same time, and boil for 1 minute to partially cook them. Using a slotted spoon, quickly remove them from the water and place in the ice water. Let them cool for about a minute, then drain through a colander and pat dry.

On a serving plate, layer the mozzarella slices, 10 basil leaves, asparagus, and peas. Drizzle with the vinaigrette to your taste and sprinkle with a little more salt and freshly cracked pepper. Serve cold or at room temperature.

NOTE: For a dairy-free/plant-based option, omit the mozzarella.

Shaved Asparagus Flatbreads

MAKES 4 SERVINGS

This makes a great dinner for Friday night when you don't want to put in a lot of effort. It also makes an elegant appetizer or even a quick lunch. Shaving asparagus into thin pieces allows it to cook quickly in the oven (and may be a super fun new way to get the kids and spouse on board with more vegetables?!). See tips on page 67 for how to store asparagus so it lasts longer.

½ pound asparagus spears

2 teaspoons extra-virgin olive oil

¼ teaspoon kosher salt

Freshly cracked black pepper to taste

4 pita breads (naan bread will also work), whole wheat preferred

½ pound fresh mozzarella cheese, sliced

2 ounces soft goat cheese, crumbled

1 clove garlic, halved

Preheat the oven to 500°F. Trim the thick, woody ends from the asparagus spears. Use a peeler to shave down the sides of asparagus, shaving them into very thin slices. Toss the shaved asparagus with the olive oil, salt, and pepper until well coated.

Place the pita breads on a baking sheet and rub with the cut side of the garlic clove. Place them in the oven and bake for 3 minutes. Remove the pitas from the oven and top evenly with the fresh mozzarella, then shaved asparagus, then the goat cheese crumbles. Bake until the cheese is melted and lightly browned on top and the pita is crisp on the edges, 8 to 9 minutes.

Let the flatbreads cool for about 5 minutes before serving.

NOTE: For a gluten-free option, opt for a cauliflower pizza crust. Cook according to package directions.

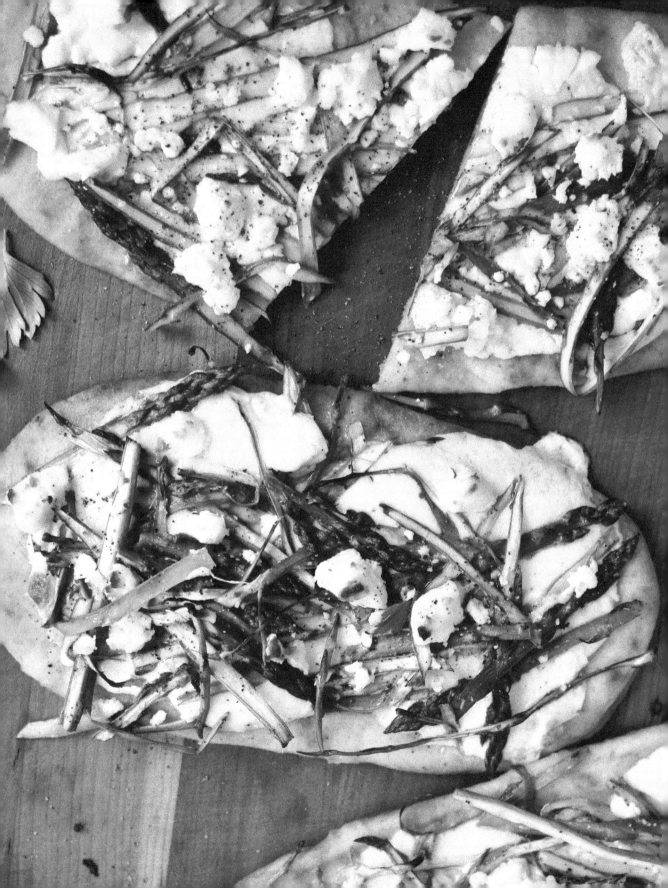

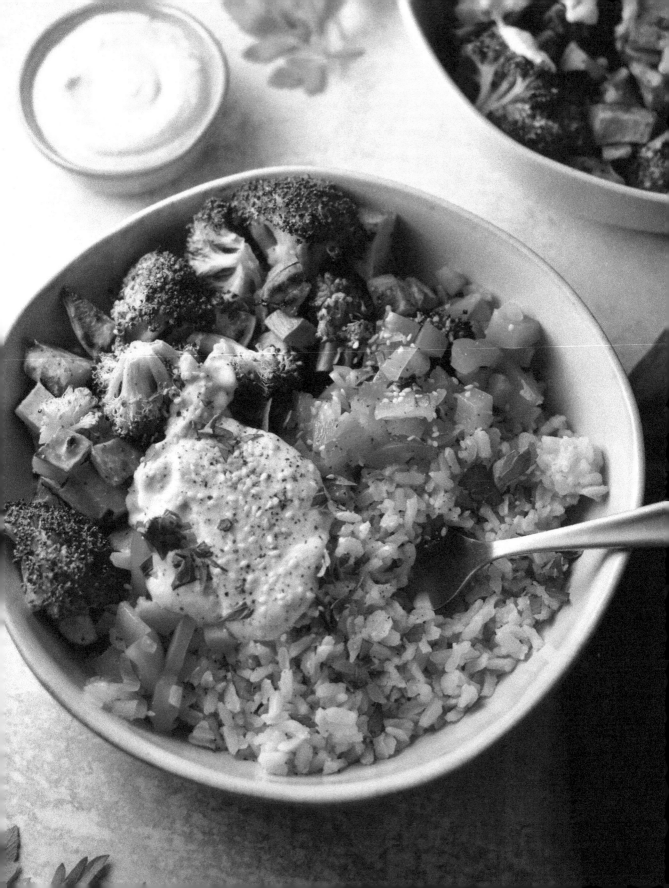

Tahini Sweet Potato Bowl

MAKES 4 SERVINGS

One of my favorite plant-based meals from thedizzycook.com, this recipe is filling and comforting and packed full of wonderful nutrients. Pair with pre-cooked rice, bulgur, or quinoa for a full meal. While sweet potatoes aren't typical ingredients in the Mediterranean region, they're known to help prevent cancer and support the immune system—which makes them a nutrient-dense choice to add to meals. If adding any other vegetables, roast them along with the broccoli or just toss them into the bowl raw.

ROASTED VEGETABLES

3 tablespoons olive oil

4 sweet potatoes,
 cut into ½-inch cubes

Kosher salt and freshly ground
 black pepper

12 ounces broccoli florets

TAHINI DRESSING

¼ cup plus 1 tablespoon tahini

1 garlic clove, minced

2 teaspoons honey

¼ cup distilled white vinegar

2 tablespoons toasted
 sesame oil

2 tablespoons olive oil

2 teaspoons ground ginger

Kosher salt

2 to 3 tablespoons cold water,
 if needed

ACCOMPANIMENTS

Hot cooked brown rice, bulgur,
 or quinoa

1 red bell pepper, chopped,
 or ¾ cup chopped carrots

3 green onions, chopped

2 tablespoons sesame seeds,
 toasted (see page 54)

To make the vegetables, preheat the oven to 425°F and line a large baking sheet with parchment paper. Toss the sweet potato cubes with 2 tablespoons olive oil, ½ teaspoon salt, and ¼ teaspoon pepper and spread them out on the baking sheet. Roast for 20 minutes. Prepare the broccoli by tossing it with the remaining 1 tablespoon olive oil, along with salt and pepper to taste.

After 20 minutes, toss the sweet potatoes and add the broccoli to the same sheet pan, spreading out the vegetables again. Continue to roast until the vegetables are browned and tender, about 20 more minutes.

While the vegetables are roasting, make the tahini dressing: In a food processor, combine the tahini, garlic, honey, vinegar, sesame oil, olive oil, ginger, and salt to taste. Turn on the machine and process, adding the water as needed, until the desired consistency is reached. Taste and see if it needs salt—some tahini brands are saltier than others. Set aside at room temperature.

To assemble, divide the warm rice among serving bowls. Divide the roasted vegetables evenly over the rice. Top each portion with the raw vegetables, tahini sauce to taste, green onions, and toasted sesame seeds. Serve right away.

Boursin Broccoli Soup

MAKES 4 TO 6 SERVINGS

If you're a big fan of broccoli-cheddar soup, this recipe is a bit more migraine-friendly, using fresh cheese rather than aged cheddar. The garlic and herbs in the cheese give the soup a Mediterranean flair. Because it is already full-flavored, using Boursin in the soup saves you the extra effort of adding lots of seasonings.

¼ cup extra-virgin olive oil

2 large shallots, chopped

2 large carrots, chopped small (about 1 cup)

¼ cup all-purpose flour

3 cups vegetable broth

1½ cups milk

1 head broccoli, chopped into florets (about 2 full cups florets)

5 ounces Boursin Garlic & Herb cheese

¾ teaspoon kosher salt, or to taste

½ teaspoon freshly ground black pepper

In a large, heavy pot (I used a 5½-quart pot), warm the olive oil over medium heat and stir in the shallots and carrots. Sauté until the vegetables are fragrant and tender, about 2 minutes. Add the flour and stir to coat the vegetables. Pour in about ½ cup of the broth and whisk until the flour gets incorporated and the mixture is smooth. Add the rest of the broth along with the milk. Bring the mixture to a low simmer and simmer until thickened, 8 to 10 minutes. Do not let the mixture boil, or the milk could curdle (especially if you're using a low-fat option).

Add the broccoli florets and cook until softened, about 5 minutes. Remove the soup from the heat, add the Boursin, salt, and pepper, and stir until smooth and creamy. Taste and adjust any seasonings.

Ladle the soup into bowls and serve hot.

NOTE: To make this a gluten-free soup, use gluten-free all-purpose flour. To make this a dairy-free soup, you could try dairy-free Boursin cheese. Although it contains "natural flavors," which can potentially point to hidden MSG, many of my Dizzy Cook readers tolerate it very well.

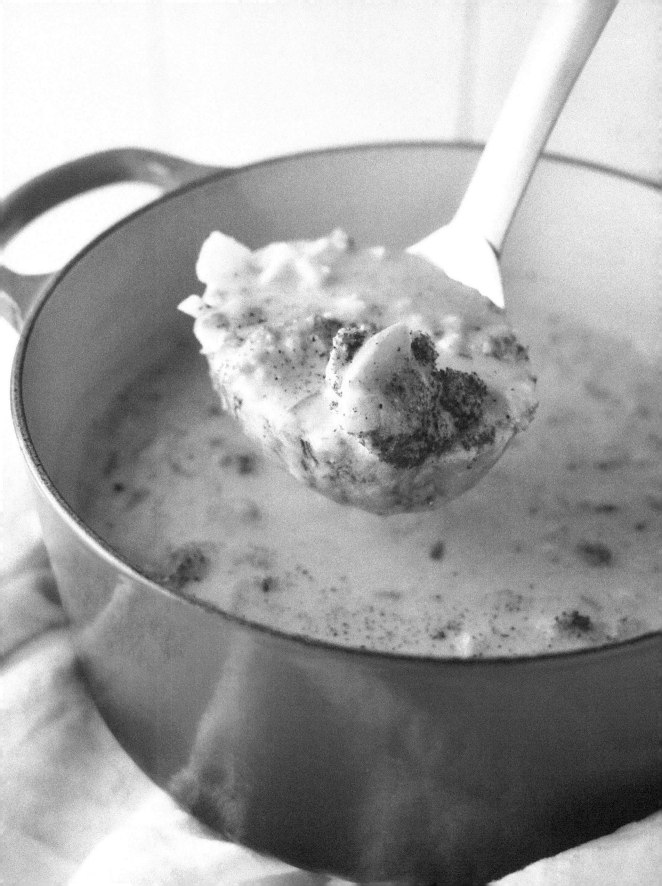

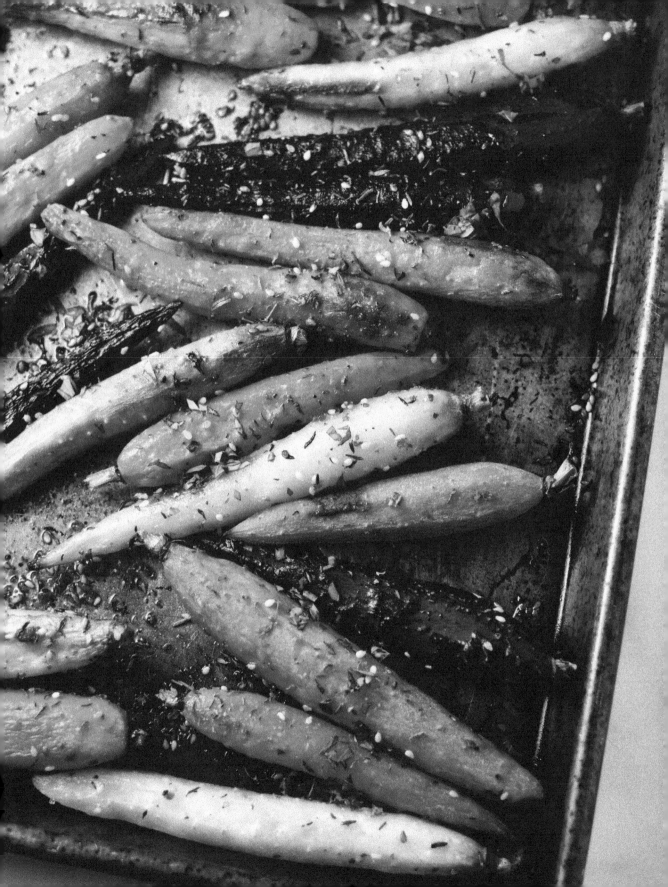

Za'atar Roasted Carrots

MAKES 4 TO 6 SIDE-DISH SERVINGS

Za'atar is a blend of spices and herbs like oregano and cumin, dried sumac, and toasted sesame seeds. It has a nutty, earthy flavor with a hint of tanginess from the sumac. It's wonderful on chicken, hummus, and roasted vegetables like these carrots. This simple side dish is delicious and easy, pairing perfectly with the Tart Cherry Grilled Steak (page 215) or grilled chicken. You can find pre-mixed za'atar at most grocery stores (Trader Joe's has it) or online, or make your own at home. Want to be super decadent? Pair this with burrata or whipped ricotta and warm bread for an appetizer that will convince your friends you are a top chef!

---

2 pounds whole carrots, peeled

2 tablespoons extra-virgin olive oil

1 teaspoon kosher salt

2½ teaspoons za'atar

1 tablespoon chopped fresh parsley

Preheat the oven to 425°F.

Toss the carrots with the olive oil, salt, and za'atar and spread evenly on a baking sheet. Roast until the carrots are lightly golden and tender, 20 to 25 minutes.

Transfer the carrots to a serving dish, sprinkle with the parsley, and serve warm.

Garlicky Roasted Green Beans

MAKES 4 TO 6 SIDE-DISH SERVINGS

A common way of preparing green beans is to sauté them, but I love roasting when I need to cook a lot at one time. They are super flavorful and don't require much effort beyond tossing with garlic and olive oil! Pair with Roasted Branzino (page 159) or chicken. French-style green beans, also known as haricots verts, are thinner than normal green beans and cook much faster. If you're using regular green beans, increase the roasting time to 15 to 18 minutes.

---

16 ounces French green beans (haricots verts), trimmed

2 tablespoons extra-virgin olive oil

2 cloves garlic, minced

½ teaspoon kosher salt

¼ teaspoon freshly ground black pepper

2 tablespoons chopped fresh parsley

Preheat the oven to 425°F.

Toss the green beans with the olive oil, garlic, salt, and pepper until coated. Arrange the beans on a baking sheet in a single layer. Roast until softened and brown in spots, 10 to 15 minutes.

Transfer the beans to a serving dish and sprinkle with the parsley. Serve warm.

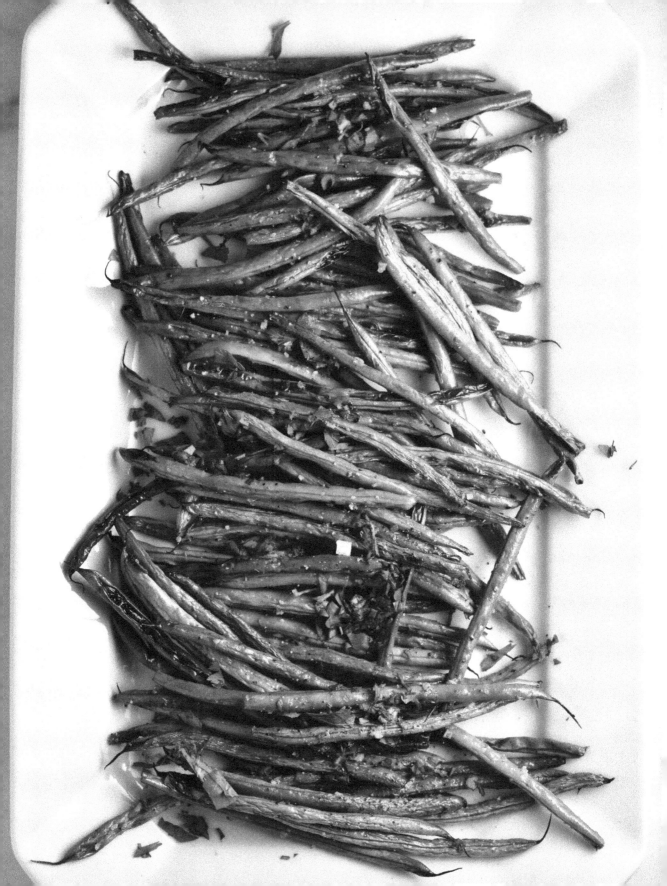

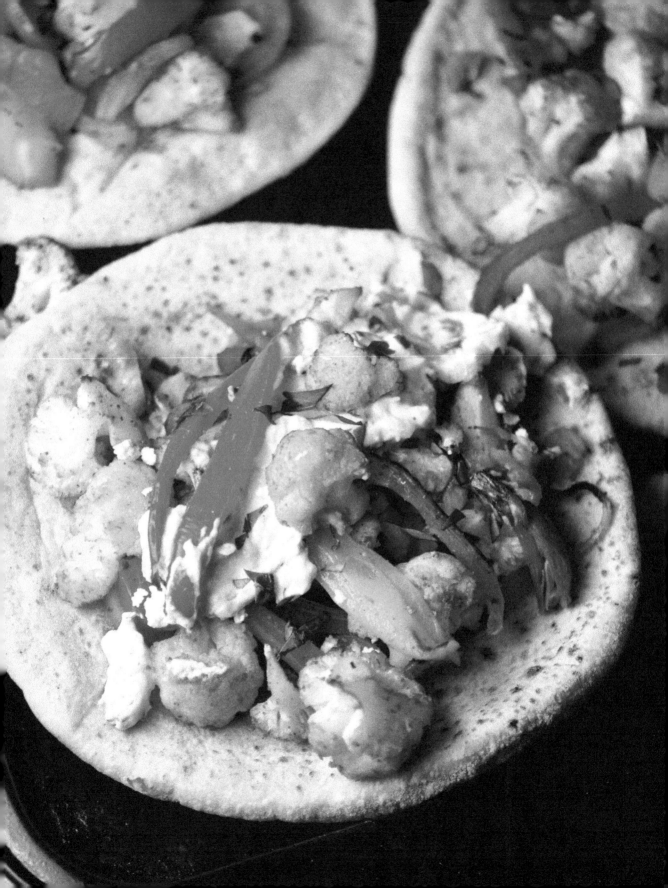

Cauliflower Pitas with Faux Tzatziki

MAKES 4 TO 6 SERVINGS

There's so much flavor in these pita sandwiches! Spiced cauliflower, peppers, and shallots are the perfect complement to the creamy sauce. Yogurt happens to be one of my personal migraine triggers, but I discovered that I could make a version of the classic garlic and cucumber sauce using cottage cheese. Once whipped, the texture is light and fluffy, and it packs even more protein than yogurt.

FILLING

1¼ pounds (20 ounces) cauliflower (about 1 large head), cut into small florets

1 small red bell pepper, sliced

1 small yellow bell pepper, sliced

2 shallots, sliced

1 tablespoon extra-virgin olive oil

1 teaspoon ground cumin

1 teaspoon paprika

½ teaspoon kosher salt

⅛ teaspoon freshly ground black pepper

FAUX TZATZIKI

1 English cucumber (unpeeled)

¾ cup cottage cheese

1 to 2 garlic cloves

1 tablespoon distilled white vinegar or lemon juice

1 tablespoon chopped fresh dill

4 pita breads

Crumbled feta cheese (optional)

Preheat the oven to 425°F.

To make the filling, in a large bowl, toss the cauliflower florets, red and yellow pepper, and shallots with the olive oil, cumin, paprika, salt, and pepper until coated. Spread in an even layer on large baking sheet and roast until softened and golden brown, 20 to 25 minutes. Remove the vegetables from the oven.

Meanwhile, make the faux tzatziki sauce: Grate the cucumber using the large holes of a box grater-shredder and place on a paper towel (you'll need about ⅔ cup). Gather the shredded cucumber in the paper towel and squeeze firmly to get out as much liquid as you can.

Place the cottage cheese in a small food processor and add the garlic to your preference (2 cloves is VERY garlicky, so you've been warned). Turn on the machine and blend until smooth. With a rubber spatula, stir in the grated cucumber, vinegar, and dill. Transfer to a bowl and refrigerate for at least 20 minutes to allow the flavors to blend.

Place the pitas on a baking sheet and put them in the oven until softened and warmed through, 3 to 5 minutes.

To assemble, divide the vegetables among the warmed pita breads and top each with a dollop of the faux tzatziki sauce. Sprinkle with feta cheese, if desired, and serve right away.

NOTE: For a dairy-free version, omit the tzatziki and cheese. For a gluten-free version, serve the vegetables on top of rice or quinoa, or folded inside a gluten-free tortilla.

PortoPizzas

MAKES 6 PIZZAS

Here, I use meaty portobello mushroom caps in place of pizza crusts for delicious individual pizzas. This is the perfect recipe for any time that you want to sneak additional veggies into your meals. It's easy to make, and using good-quality toppings takes this to the next level. I used Nomato Sauce (page 96) for this recipe, but you could substitute your favorite marinara.

Olive oil, if needed

6 portobello mushroom caps

1 cup Nomato Sauce (page 96) or prepared marinara sauce

½ cup fresh spinach leaves

One 8-ounce ball fresh mozzarella cheese, sliced into ¼-inch rounds

Handful of fresh basil leaves

Kosher salt and freshly ground black pepper

Preheat the oven to 425°F. Spray or brush a large, rimmed baking sheet with olive oil or line it with parchment paper.

Carefully wipe the outside of the portobello caps using a damp paper towel to remove any lingering dirt—do not run them under water, which will make them mushy. Turn over the mushroom caps and, using the side of a small spoon, carefully remove the inner ribs and thick inner stem. Set the mushrooms top side down on the prepared baking sheet.

Divide the sauce evenly among the portobello cups. Top each with a few spinach leaves, then add small slices of mozzarella. Bake until the portobello caps have softened and the cheese is melted and light brown, 8 to 10 minutes. Top each with a few fresh basil leaves and a sprinkle of salt and pepper to taste. Serve warm.

NOTE: For dairy-free/plant-based "pizzas," omit the cheese. Many dairy-free cheeses contain additives and high-glutamate ingredients like nutritional yeast, so I don't often recommend them as a substitute for dairy cheese unless they have been ruled out as a personal trigger.

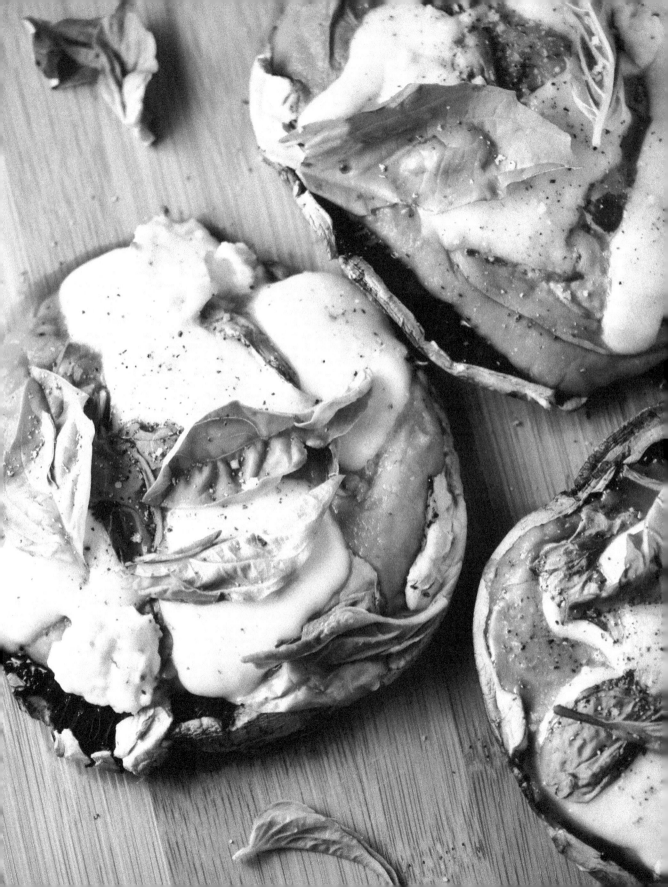

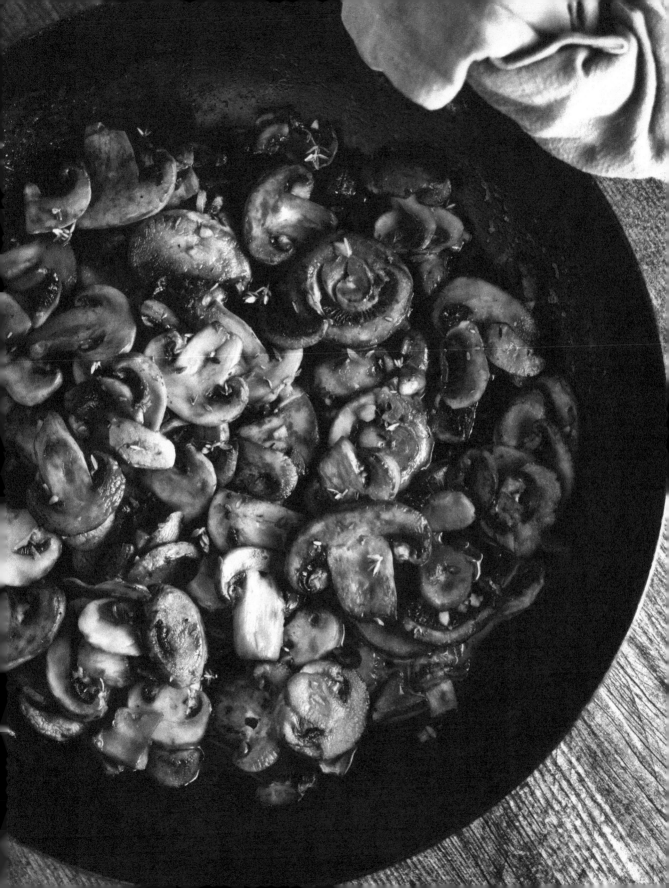

Alicia's Favorite Mushrooms

MAKES 4 TO 6 SIDE-DISH SERVINGS

Delicious and creamy, with just the perfect amount of fresh thyme, I make these savory mushrooms about once a week to top chicken, steak, or toasted bread with an egg. These were the star side dish of Thanksgiving 2021, which will live in infamy as the year we gave up turkey in lieu of grilling steaks. Although not a common Mediterranean ingredient, I love to add 2 teaspoons of coconut aminos just before adding the cream. It will sizzle and cook down but adds an extra layer of flavor.

---

1 tablespoon extra-virgin olive oil

16 ounces sliced button or cremini mushrooms

4 garlic cloves, minced

4 teaspoons heavy cream

1 to 2 teaspoons fresh thyme leaves, or substitute chopped fresh rosemary

Kosher salt and freshly ground black pepper to taste

In a large skillet, warm the olive oil over medium-high heat. Working in batches, add a layer of the mushroom slices, making sure to not crowd the pan. Let them cook, undisturbed, until a deep, caramelized brown on one side, 2 to 3 minutes, then flip the mushrooms to brown on the other side, stirring occasionally with a wooden spoon. Push the cooked mushrooms to the sides of the pan if possible, or transfer them to a plate and cook the next batch in the same manner until all of the mushrooms are cooked.

Once all mushrooms are browned and softened, return them to the center of the pan. Reduce the heat to medium and add the cream and thyme leaves. Cook until the cream has thickened and coated the mushrooms, 1 to 2 minutes. Season with kosher salt and pepper to taste. Serve warm.

NOTE: For a dairy-free option, use coconut cream or oat milk to replace the heavy cream.

Nomato Sauce

MAKES ABOUT 2 CUPS

Food triggers can be tricky to navigate when living with migraine. A huge staple of the Mediterranean diet is tomatoes, but I do find a few of my migraine friends to be sensitive to them in varying levels. If that's you—don't worry! You will love this faux marinara sauce that uses beets and carrots to create a savory addition to pizzas or pasta. It sounds weird, but it just works. I like to give people an equal opportunity to enjoy dishes they love, despite what their personal triggers are. And while I'm personally not sensitive to tomatoes, I still love this sauce! It's a great way to get extra vegetables into your meal, and you can't taste the beets. Use it for a pizza sauce, pasta sauce, dipping sauce, and more.

1 tablespoon extra-virgin olive oil

3 garlic cloves, minced

1 shallot, chopped

2½ cups finely chopped carrots

⅔ cup chopped cooked red beets

1 teaspoon dried Mediterranean oregano

1 tablespoon chopped fresh basil

1 tablespoon distilled white vinegar

1½ cups vegetable broth

½ teaspoon kosher salt

Freshly ground black pepper

In a large sauté pan, warm the olive oil over medium-high heat. Add the garlic, shallot, carrots, and beets and cook, stirring frequently, until carrots have softened, about 7 minutes. Add the oregano, basil, vinegar, and broth. Bring the liquid to a simmer and cook until the carrots are very soft (this is why they need to be chopped small, so they cook quickly), another 10 minutes.

Transfer the mixture into a high-speed blender (or use an immersion blender) to blend until the sauce is very smooth. Serve right away, or pour into a Mason jar and let cool before sealing. This sauce will keep in the refrigerator for up to 1 week or in the freezer for up to 4 months.

TIP: Mediterranean oregano is sometimes simply labeled as "oregano" in stores. Just don't confuse it with Mexican oregano, which has a different flavor.

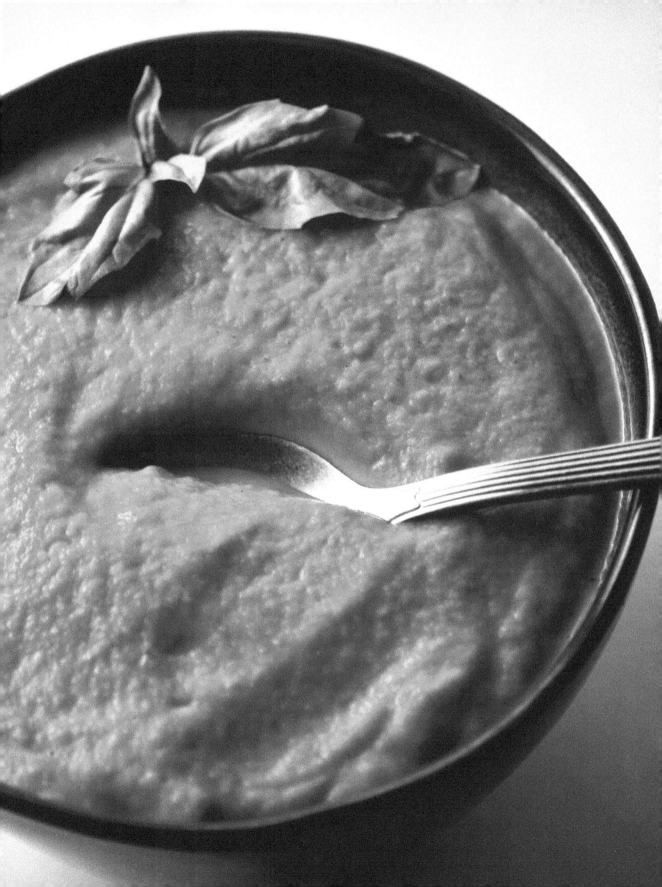

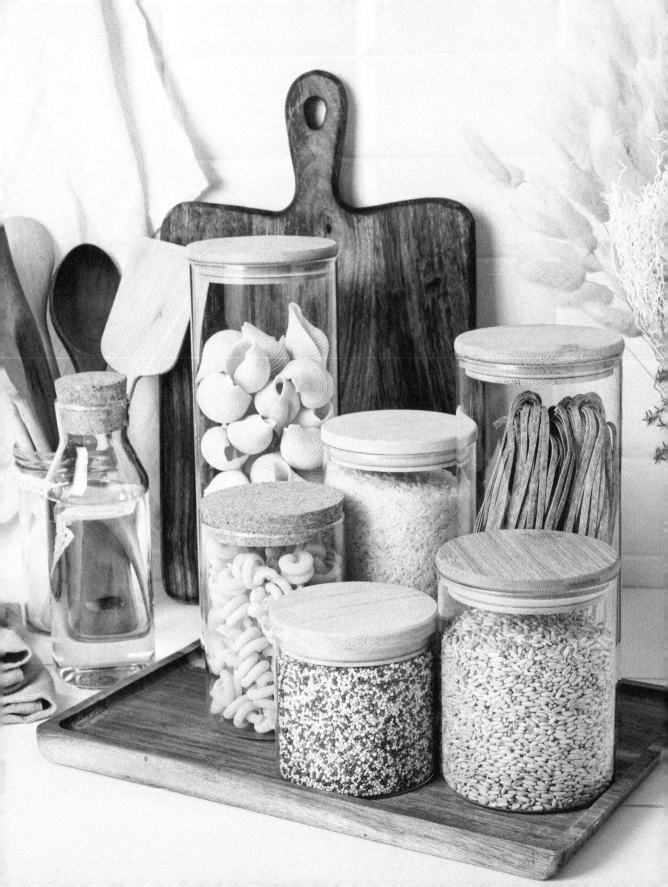

GRAINS

For more recipes featuring grains, see the index.

THE BENEFITS OF WHOLE GRAINS

Whole grains are an important part of Mediterranean cuisine. They are a rich source of B vitamins and minerals. Conversely, refined grains are devoid of practically all nutrients and polyphenols because the nutrient-packed bran layer and cereal germ has been removed. Because of the lack of fiber, consuming refined grain products (like white bread or white rice) causes a blood glucose spike, just like eating sugar.

Wheat is one of the most widely produced grains in the world. FARRO refers to three wheat species (spelt, einkorn, and emmer) that are sold dried, and cooked in water until soft. Farro is an ancient grain, and has featured in Italian cuisine for centuries. Farro is sold as whole (with the nutritious bran intact), semi-pearled (the bran partially removed), and pearled (the bran stripped completely). BULGUR is made from cracked parboiled whole wheat grains. It is used in Mediterranean and Middle Eastern cuisine. Bulgur does not require cooking, and just needs to be soaked in water, but can be cooked in some dishes. It is sold in a variety of grinds: fine, medium, coarse, and extra coarse. COUSCOUS are granules made from crushed durum wheat or barley.

RICE was first cultivated in the Yangtze basin in China. With migration and trade, rice spread all over the world and is used in many different cuisines. Brown rice is the whole grain form of rice, while white rice is the polished form. Red rice is a species of rice colored red by antioxidant anthrocyanins in the bran. Black (or purple) rice contains very high levels of anthrocyanins in the bran layer.

QUINOA is from South America, not the Mediterranean region, but it is a grain with fabulous nutritional properties, and should be part of your diet. There are three types: white, red, and black. Quinoa is packed with fiber, manganese, copper, iron, and folate, as well as two antioxidant flavonoids called quercetin and kaempferol. It should be rinsed several times before cooking to remove the saponins, which have a bitter aftertaste.

When choosing pasta, look for pasta made from whole wheat. Healthy options (which have a slightly different texture and taste) include pasta made from edamame, chickpeas, and quinoa.

When making bread-based dishes, choose breads made from whole-wheat flour or graham flour, a coarse-ground whole-wheat flour.

COOKING WITH WHOLE GRAINS

Whole grains are a great staple for creating filling salads or sides while also adding a lot of nutrition to meals, as Dr. Beh points out. Some of my favorites that can be easily found are quinoa, rice, couscous, farro, and a variety of different pasta shapes. For these recipes, we encourage buying whole wheat pastas or even chickpea pasta, which has just a touch more protein than standard grain-based pasta.

It's important to note couscous and farro are not gluten free, so if you have a sensitivity, brown rice or quinoa make great substitutes in recipes. I buy most grains at Trader Joe's for the good price, but a lot of grocery stores also have a bulk section with a wider variety. This is where you might spot less common grain varieties like bulgur or buckwheat.

Whole-grain bread is also a delicious, healthy base for Mediterranean-style meals. Top it with fresh cheese and seasonal vegetables for an easy meal.

Sweet Potato & Grain Salad with Parsley Vinaigrette

MAKES 4 TO 6 SIDE-DISH SERVINGS

While regular potatoes and bulgur are more typical of what you might see in a classic Mediterranean dish, I like the addition of sweet potatoes and quinoa in this grain-based salad for a vibrant color, increased protein content, and enhanced nutrients. This is a great meal for any time of year. The roasted sweet potatoes and cauliflower are complemented by a parsley vinaigrette. Serve as a vegetarian meal or with grilled chicken or Tart Cherry Grilled Steak (page 214).

SALAD

3 cups sweet potatoes, diced (2 to 3 small sweet potatoes)

1 tablespoon extra-virgin olive oil

Kosher salt and freshly ground black pepper

12 ounces cauliflower florets

PARSLEY VINAIGRETTE

1 cup fresh parsley leaves

1/3 cup extra-virgin olive oil

1 clove garlic

1 teaspoon honey

1/4 teaspoon kosher salt

1 cup broth

1 cup water

1 cup quinoa, rinsed

4 green onions, ends trimmed and chopped

Preheat the oven to 425°F. Line a large, rimmed baking sheet with parchment paper.

To make the salad, place the sweet potatoes on the prepared pan and drizzle with olive oil and add salt and pepper to taste. Toss to coat and bake for 20 minutes.

Add the cauliflower florets to the pan and toss well. Bake until the vegetables are soft and light brown, about 20 more minutes

While the vegetables are roasting, make the vinaigrette: In a small food processor, blend together the parsley leaves, olive oil, garlic, honey, and salt until smooth. Set aside.

In a saucepan over medium-high heat, warm the broth and water. Once simmering, add the quinoa, cover, and cook over low heat until the liquid is absorbed and quinoa is light and fluffy, 15 to 20 minutes.

In a serving bowl, toss the roasted vegetables, green onion, and cooked quinoa together. Add half of the vinaigrette and toss well. Taste and add more dressing, if desired. Serve warm or at room temperature.

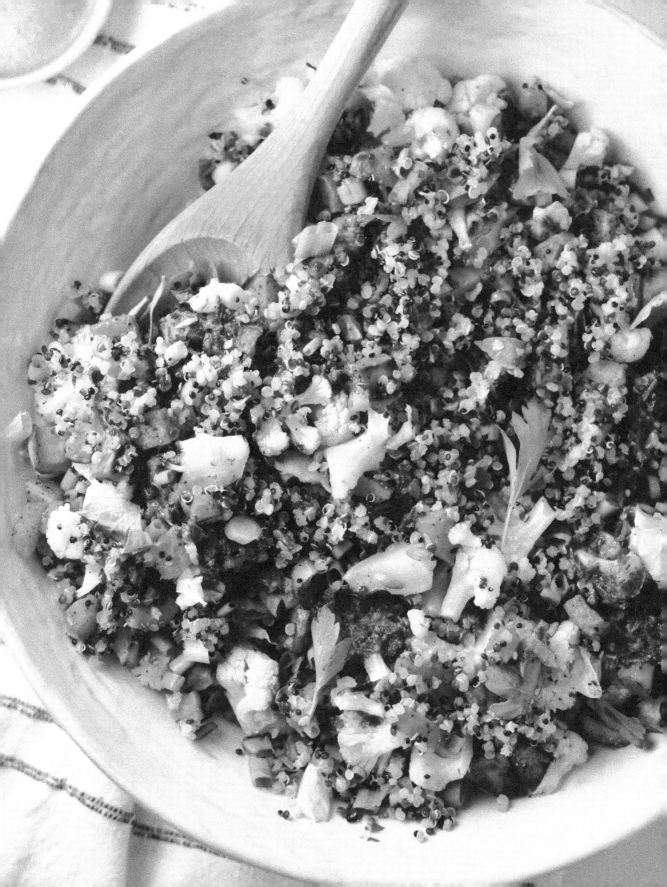

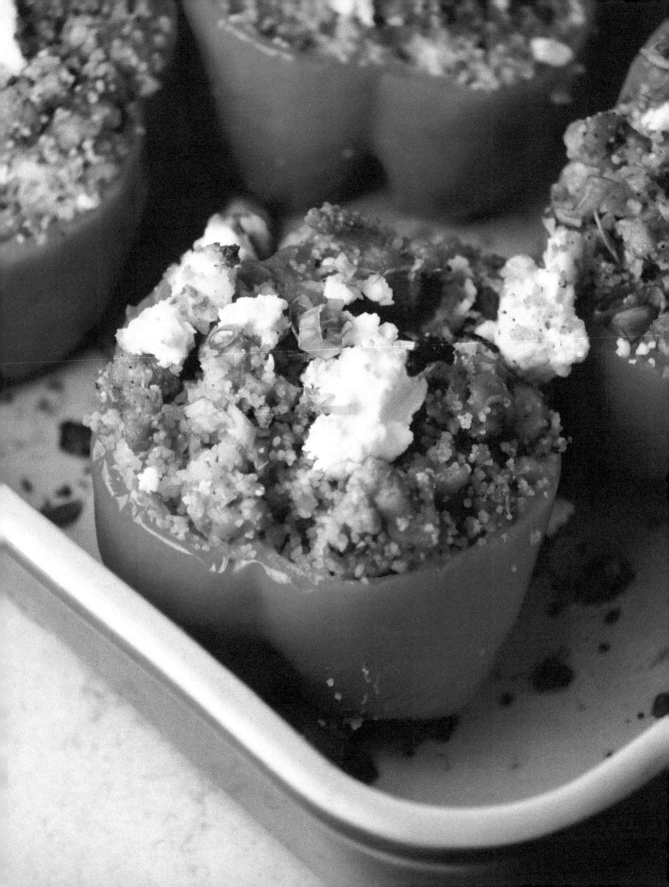

Couscous & Lamb Stuffed Peppers

MAKES 6 STUFFED PEPPERS

This recipe is so versatile! I often substitute ground beef or chicken for the lamb. You could also turn it into a vegetarian dish with your favorite leftover roasted vegetables. Store this in the fridge up to three days for a great leftover meal. When buying couscous for this recipe, be sure to buy the durum wheat type, which is small and grainy, and not Israeli couscous, which is large and round.

---

6 bell peppers, red or yellow recommended

1 cup vegetable broth

1 tablespoon extra-virgin olive oil, plus more for sautéing

1 cup durum wheat couscous

1 pound ground lamb

1 shallot, chopped

1 garlic clove, minced

Kosher salt and pepper

1 teaspoon dried Mediterranean oregano

¼ cup soft goat cheese or feta

Preheat the oven to 400°F. Spray or brush a 9-by-13-inch baking pan with olive oil.

Cut the top stem off bell peppers and remove any seeds. Arrange the peppers, cut side up, in the prepared baking pan.

In a saucepan, bring the broth to a simmer and add the 1 tablespoon olive oil. Stir in the couscous, cover with a lid, and turn off the heat. Allow the mixture to stand for 10 minutes. Uncover and fluff the grains with a fork.

In a large skillet, sauté the lamb over medium heat until cooked through, 5 to 6 minutes. Add the shallot and garlic and cook until softened, 1 to 2 minutes. Add the couscous and oregano and season with salt and pepper to taste.

Spoon the lamb-couscous mixture into the bell pepper cavities, dividing evenly. Top evenly with cheese, cover with foil, and bake for 20 to 25 minutes. Uncover and bake until lightly brown on top, about 5 minutes. Serve warm.

NOTE: For a gluten-free dish, replace the couscous with brown rice. For a dairy-free dish, omit the cheese.

Turmeric-Ginger Rice

MAKES 4 SIDE-DISH SERVINGS

As a vestibular migraine patient, I often think about quick and easy meals to prepare when I'm not feeling my best. This is great by itself on attack days, or serve this rice alongside chicken, meatballs, fish, or roasted vegetables for a full meal. To make this dish a little more festive, stir in a handful of pomegranate seeds after cooking the rice.

---

1 tablespoon extra-virgin olive oil

1 cup brown rice

1 teaspoon ground turmeric

½ teaspoon ground ginger

2 shallots, chopped (about ½ cup)

2 cups vegetable broth

Fresh cilantro springs for garnish, optional

In a saucepan, warm the olive oil over medium heat. Add the rice and stir with a wooden spoon to coat the grains with the oil. Allow the rice to brown a bit, releasing a nutty flavor, 2 to 3 minutes. Stir in the turmeric and ginger until the rice is well coated. Add the shallots and then stir in the broth. Bring to a simmer over medium-high heat.

When the liquid is simmering, cover the pan, reduce the heat to low, and cook until all liquid is absorbed, about 40 minutes. Remove from the heat and let stand, covered, for a few minutes and then fluff the rice with a fork. Serve warm garnished with fresh cilantro sprigs, if desired.

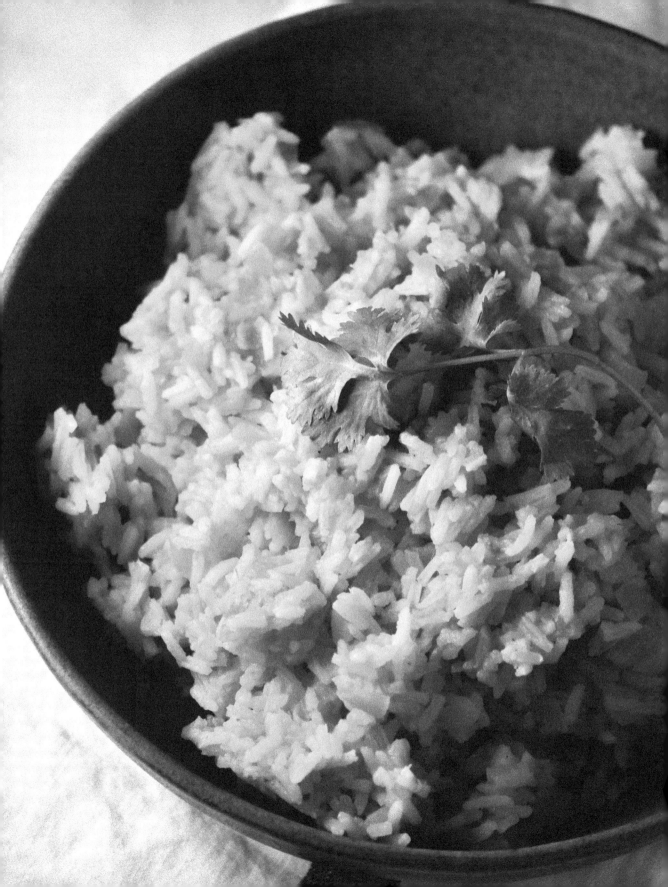

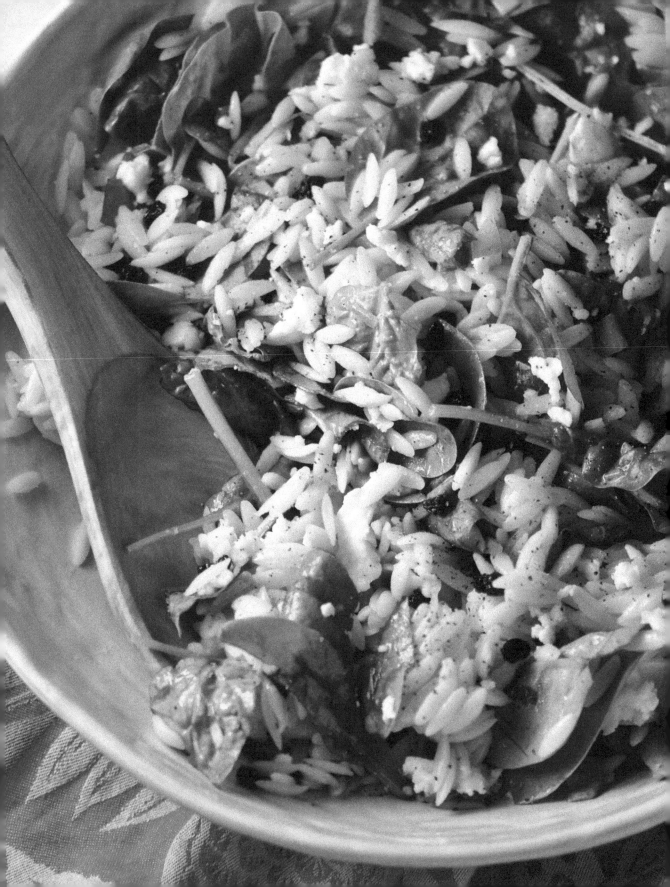

Spinach Orzo Salad

MAKES 4 TO 6 SIDE-DISH SERVINGS

This light pasta salad is perfect for lunches or summer cookouts. I actually pack this for a plane lunch (without the cheese) if I'm trying to watch my migraine trigger load while traveling. Without the cheese, it keeps well for a few hours unrefrigerated. Dried currants or pomegranate seeds, which are high in antioxidants, add a touch of sweetness to the salty and savory pasta. If you are using a very salty feta, you may want to scale back on the added salt to roughly ¼ teaspoon.

DRESSING

¼ cup chopped shallots

1 teaspoon honey

1 tablespoon Dijon mustard

2 teaspoons distilled white vinegar

¼ cup olive oil

SALAD

8 ounces dried orzo

1 to 2 cups fresh spinach leaves

¼ cup dried currants (sulfite-free) or fresh pomegranate seeds

2 ounces feta or fresh goat cheese

½ teaspoon kosher salt

¼ teaspoon fresh black pepper

To make the dressing, in a small bowl, combine the shallots, honey, Dijon, and vinegar and whisk until blended. While whisking, slowly add the olive oil until smooth and well blended. Set aside.

To make the salad, prepare the orzo according to the package directions. Once cooked, drain through a colander and run under cold water to stop the cooking. Drain again well.

Add the drained orzo to a large bowl and add the spinach and currants. Add ¼ cup of the dressing and toss well, adding additional dressing to taste (save any remaining dressing for another use). Add the feta or goat cheese and season with salt and pepper. Serve cold or at room temperature.

NOTE: For a dairy-free/plant-based option, omit the cheese. For a gluten-free dish, try using Jovial's cassava orzo.

Rustic Toasts with Shaved Vegetables & Whipped Goat Cheese

MAKES 4 TOASTS

Can y'all tell I'm really into shaved vegetables? Seriously though, you could use almost any thinly shaved vegetable for this quick snack or lunch. Shaved vegetable salads are popular all over the Mediterranean region for good reason: They're a great way to get extra vegetables into your meals. And when they're sliced this thinly, no cooking is required.

4 ounces plain soft goat cheese

1 ounce cream cheese

4 slices rustic whole-grain bread

1 large carrot

1 small zucchini

Za'atar seasoning

Fresh chives

Sea salt and freshly cracked black pepper

Extra-virgin olive oil

4 soft-boiled eggs for serving, optional

In a food processor, combine the goat cheese with cream cheese and a pinch of salt. Blend until light and smooth, stopping to scrape down the sides as needed.

Toast the bread until lightly brown on both sides. Spread one side of each bread slice with the cheese, dividing evenly.

Using a vegetable peeler, shave the carrots and zucchini into very thin strips. Pile the strips on top of the cheese-topped toasts, dividing the vegetables evenly.

Sprinkle each toast with za'atar, chives, sea salt, and pepper to taste. Drizzle with olive oil and serve right away, with halved soft-boiled eggs, if desired.

NOTE: For a dairy-free option, use Artichoke Hummus (page 125) as the base, instead of the cheese.

TIP: Don't care for goat cheese? Try using whipped ricotta or fresh burrata as a substitute.

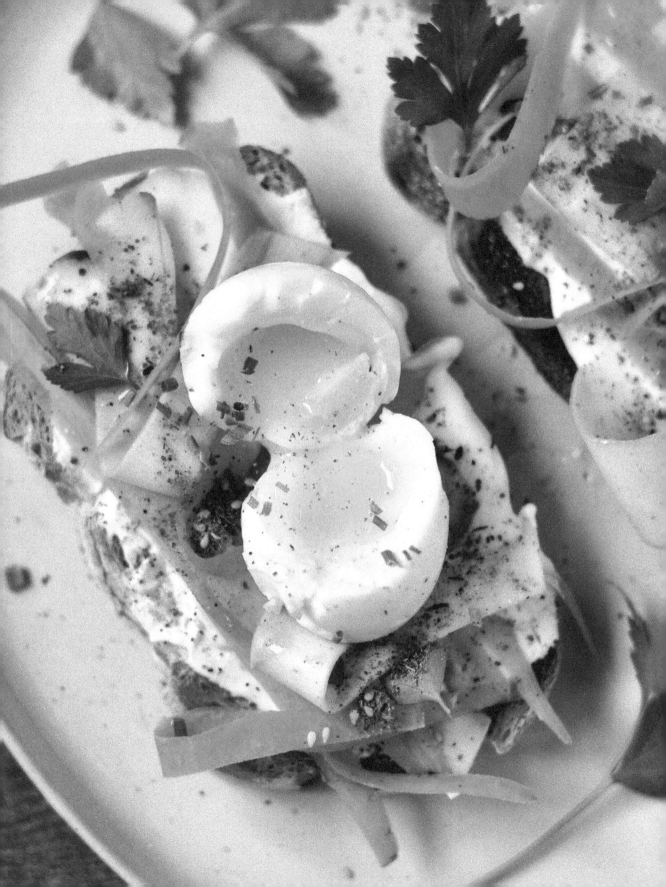

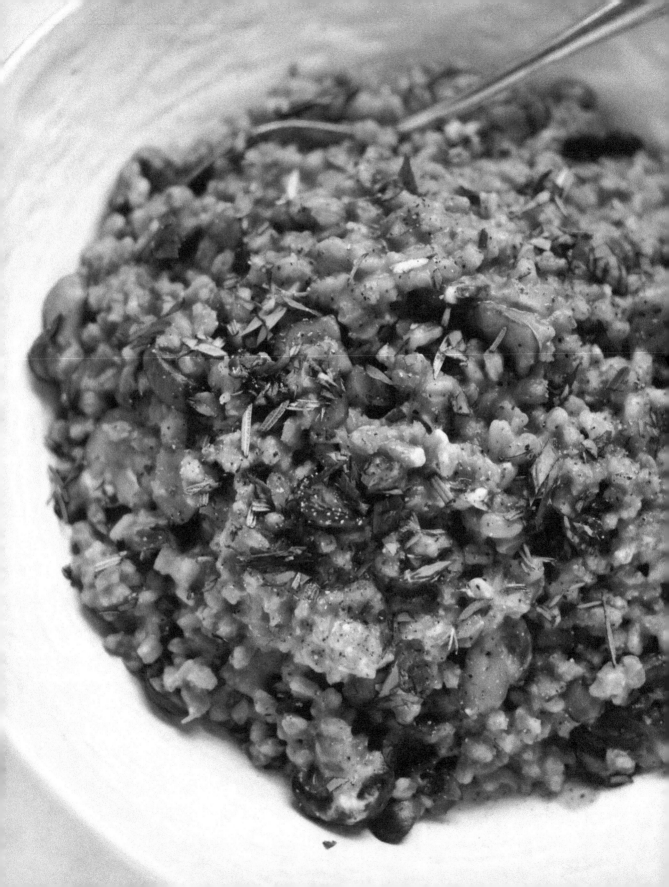

Mushroom Farroto

MAKES 4 SIDE-DISH SERVINGS

This dish is like risotto, but it's much easier because you don't need to stir it constantly. And, because it's made with whole grains, it is more nutritious. Mixed with creamy goat cheese and rosemary, this cozy meal can stand alone. Add a touch of truffle oil for extra decadence. Quick-cooking farro is also known as pearled farro and cooks in about half the time compared to whole farro. While both will taste good in this recipe, the cooking times given are meant for the quick-cooking type.

2 teaspoons extra-virgin olive oil

⅓ cup chopped shallots

10 ounces white mushrooms, sliced

3 garlic cloves, minced

1½ cups quick-cooking (pearled) farro

1 tablespoon minced fresh rosemary

3¾ cups vegetable broth

2 ounces soft goat cheese

1 tablespoon chopped fresh parsley

In a saucepan, warm the olive oil over medium-high heat. Add the shallots and cook until softened, about 1 minute. Add the mushrooms and sauté, stirring with a wooden spoon, until they start to brown and soften, 3 to 4 minutes. Stir in the garlic and then the farro. Cook, stirring, until the farro becomes slightly toasted, about 1 minute. Add the rosemary and vegetable broth.

Turn the heat to high and bring the liquid just to a boil. Cover the pan and reduce the heat to medium-low. Simmer gently for 10 to 15 minutes.

Uncover the pan and simmer until the liquid is mostly absorbed and the mixture is thick and creamy, 5 to 10 minutes.

Remove the pan from the heat and stir in the goat cheese until fully incorporated and creamy. Top with parsley and serve warm.

NOTE: For a dairy-free/plant-based option, omit the goat cheese.

Roasted Cauliflower & Saffron Pasta

MAKES 4 MAIN-DISH OR 6 SIDE-DISH SERVINGS

Any time my mom spots cauliflower in my fridge, she asks, "Oh, are you making that pasta?!" Roasted cauliflower adds a buttery, delicious flavor that pairs wonderfully with saffron. Saffron threads can be expensive, but it doesn't take much to add a ton of flavor. If it's out of your price range, try ground turmeric instead in the same amount. While it won't have the same Spanish flavor that is most often found in paella, it does pack some anti-inflammatory power.

CAULIFLOWER

16 ounces fresh cauliflower florets

Extra-virgin olive oil

Kosher salt and freshly ground black pepper

PASTA

⅓ cup panko breadcrumbs

⅓ cup chopped fresh parsley

12 ounces pasta shells or penne, whole wheat or chickpea recommended

1 tablespoon extra-virgin olive oil

⅓ cup chopped shallots

1 garlic clove, minced

½ teaspoon saffron threads

¼ cup heavy cream

¼ cup feta cheese (try goat cheese or cream cheese for a low-sodium option)

Preheat the oven to 425°F. Line a large, rimmed baking sheet with parchment paper.

Spread the cauliflower florets in an even layer on the prepared pan, breaking up any large ones. Toss with 2 to 3 teaspoons olive oil, and salt and pepper to taste until well coated. Roast until softened and golden brown, 20 to 25 minutes. Set aside but keep the oven on.

Pour the panko onto a small baking sheet and toast in the oven for 1 to 2 minutes, watching carefully to make sure it doesn't burn. Add the parsley, mix well, and set aside.

Bring a large pot of salted water to a boil and cook pasta according to package directions. Reserve about 1 cup of the pasta water and drain the pasta through a colander.

In a large sauté pan, over medium heat, warm the 1 tablespoon olive oil. Add the shallots and sauté until softened, about 1 minute. Add the garlic and saffron, continuing to stir with a wooden spoon. Add the cream and bring to a simmer. Add the pasta and toss with the sauce. The pasta should turn a yellow color from the saffron. If the mixture needs a little more creaminess, stir in the reserved pasta water a few tablespoons at a time until the desired consistency is reached. Add the roasted cauliflower and cheese and toss well. Top with the panko-parsley mixture. Divide the pasta among serving bowls and serve warm.

TIP: For a dairy-free dish, use unsweetened oat milk instead of cream and omit the feta cheese.

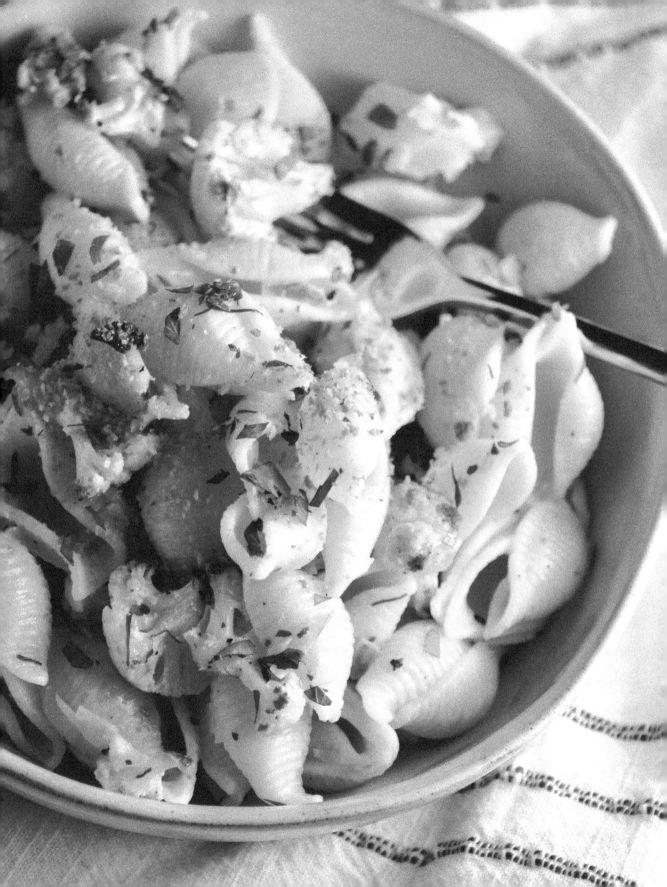

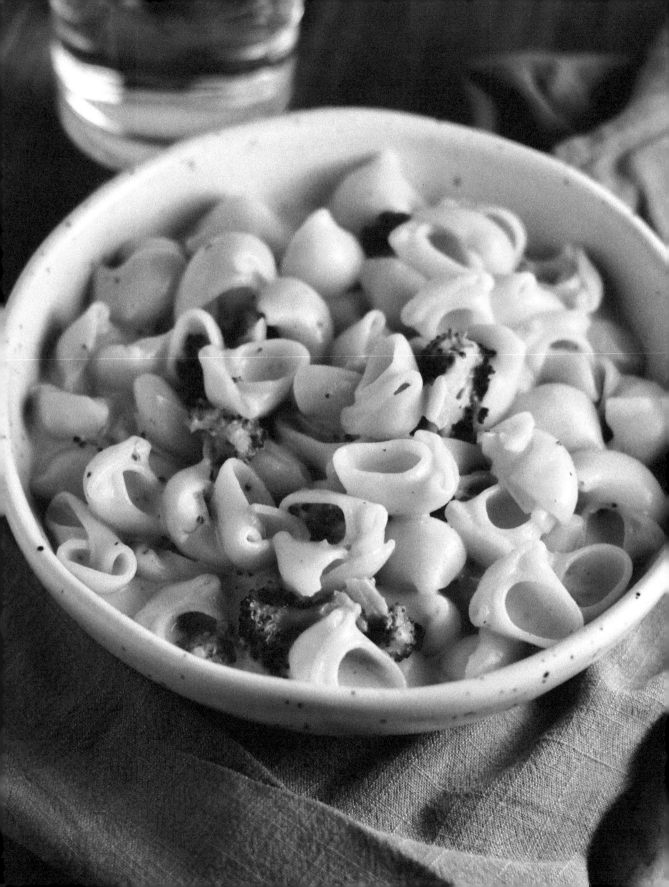

One-Pot Creamy Broccoli Mac & Cheese

MAKES 4 SERVINGS

One of the ultimate fan-favorite recipes from *The Dizzy Cook* cookbook is baked mac and cheese. When I first started a migraine diet, there were no recipes without aged cheese available and I knew there had to be a way to recreate the classic. Although this recipe isn't typically Mediterranean, I couldn't help but add one of the best comfort foods to the book that's easy to make on your bad days. You'll want a good quality American cheese, which is a combination of young Colby and young cheddar and is great for melting. Brands I like include Boar's Head, Andrew and Everett, and Horizon. If you'd like to make this with a Mediterranean twist, use an equal amount of soft goat cheese instead of American—it will be just as creamy, but with a stronger flavor.

12 ounces dry pasta shells, like pipe rigate, whole wheat or chickpea recommended

2 cups milk

2 cups low-sodium vegetable broth

1 cup water

2 cups broccoli florets, torn into very small pieces

2 garlic cloves, minced

½ teaspoon kosher salt, plus more to taste

¼ teaspoon dry mustard powder

5 ounces good-quality American cheese, shredded

Freshly ground black pepper

In a large saucepan, stir together the dry pasta shells, milk, broth, water, broccoli florets, garlic, and salt. Set the pan over high heat and bring the liquid to a boil, stirring frequently (don't forget to continue to stir to prevent the mixture from burning or boiling over). Continue to boil until the pasta is cooked and the sauce has thickened, 10 to 12 minutes. Stir in the mustard powder, cheese, and pepper to taste until the cheese has fully melted and the sauce becomes very creamy. Serve warm, adding more salt as needed.

This recipe stores and reheats very well, even microwaved. Mix in a splash of milk or broth when reheating if it needs more creaminess to the sauce.

NOTE: For a gluten-free option, choose a good-quality, gluten-free pasta instead of wheat pasta.

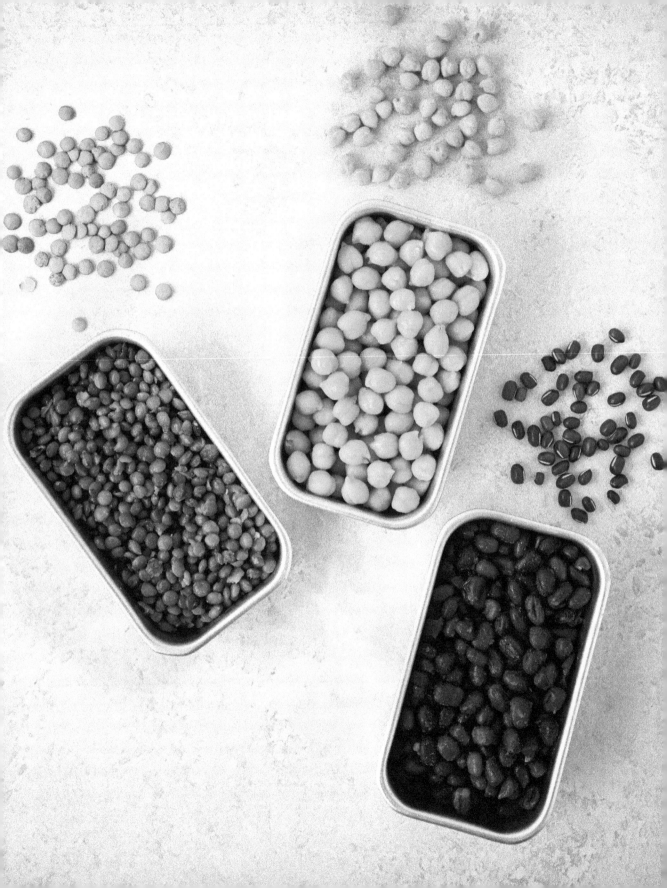

LEGUMES

For more recipes featuring legumes, see the index.

THE BENEFITS OF LEGUMES

Legumes are plants that produce pods that contain seeds, and include beans, soybeans, peas, and lentils. Legumes are a rich source of polyphenols, fiber, B vitamins, copper, zinc, and iron.

LENTILS are lens-shaped seeds used extensively in the Mediterranean region. Lentils are categorized by color, and include brown (most widely eaten), green, yellow and red, and black (or beluga).

GARBANZO BEANS (chickpeas) are a key ingredient in Mediterranean cuisine. While hummus and falafel immediately come to mind, garbanzo beans are also used to make flatbreads, salads, stews, and much more.

WHITE BEANS aren't really Mediterranean but are highly nutritious. There are several varieties of white beans, including Navy, lima, white kidney, runner, marrow, and great northern beans. White beans contain high amounts of phosphatidylserine, a fatty substance that forms the cellular membrane.

BLACK BEANS feature more in Latin American cuisine, but they can be easily incorporated into a Mediterranean-style diet. They are also called turtle beans because of their hard shell. Black beans are very nutritious, and their dense meaty texture makes them a popular addition to vegetarian foods.

ENGLISH PEAS are fiber- and nutrient-rich legumes, but what makes peas unique is the high protein content.

SHOPPING FOR LEGUMES

High in fiber and a good source of vegetarian protein, beans and legumes are easy to cook with and an inexpensive addition to any meal. For these recipes, I use canned beans because I know that cooking with migraine is already difficult, and often, we don't want to go through extra steps before even starting to make the meal.

CANNED BEANS are pre-cooked and stored in water. Be sure to look for ones without sodium added, as many brands add hefty amounts. From a texture and taste standpoint, I find dried and soaked garbanzo beans to be really great for falafels and hummus, but from a cooking with migraine perspective, it is much easier to use canned. Feel free to substitute the soaked versions for canned in these recipes! If you're just using them for soups, I like to go with the canned versions because you can't tell a difference.

YELLOW AND RED LENTILS are used a lot because they cook quickly and have a great sweet and nutty taste that pairs well with Mediterranean flavors. Puy lentils come from the French region Le Puy and have a peppery taste that pairs really well with fish or chicken sausage. You can substitute these for green lentils, but they won't have quite the same flavor. Lentils do not require soaking but should be rinsed before using. Lentils are widely found at most health food stores or can be purchased in bulk. They are a great pantry staples—perfect for a quick meal without a lot of ingredients.

English peas are best bought fresh, but frozen works in some cases. I prefer using fresh peas for salads, where you want the texture to be soft but not mushy. With frozen peas it is really difficult to control the texture, so they're best in dishes mixed with grains or pastas.

Siesta Salad

MAKES 4 TO 6 SIDE-DISH SERVINGS

I'm a Texan at heart and I can't possibly do a bean salad recipe without making it a little bit like home! I typically call this my "fiesta" salad, but since we're Med-themed, "siesta" fits perfectly. And anyone with a migraine disorder could use a few siestas! This salad is packed with great protein from the beans and lots of vegetables, making it both healthy and delicious. The smoked paprika makes this recipe a perfect pairing for burgers or any outdoor picnics. It also travels well! Garbanzo beans also will work as a substitute for black beans if you're a fan of them.

4 ears of corn, shucked

1 teaspoon extra-virgin olive oil

Kosher salt and freshly ground black pepper

3 green onions, chopped

One 15-ounce can black beans, rinsed and drained

½ cup chopped yellow bell pepper

1 cup chopped red bell pepper

½ teaspoon kosher salt

¼ teaspoon smoked paprika

Preheat a grill or stove-top grill pan to medium-high heat. Brush the corn with the olive oil and sprinkle lightly with salt and pepper. Grill the corn, turning every 2 minutes or when some of the corn is slightly charred, until cooked on all sides, 7 to 8 minutes total.

Place a small bowl upside down in a larger bowl. Balance the end of one grilled corn ear on the bowl and hold onto the other end securely. Slide a chef's knife down the cob so the kernels fall into the larger bowl. Repeat with the remaining corn ears (you'll have 2 to 3 cups total). Remove the inner bowl.

Add the green onions, black beans, bell peppers, ½ teaspoon kosher salt, and the smoked paprika and toss well. Taste and adjust any seasonings. Serve cold or at room temperature.

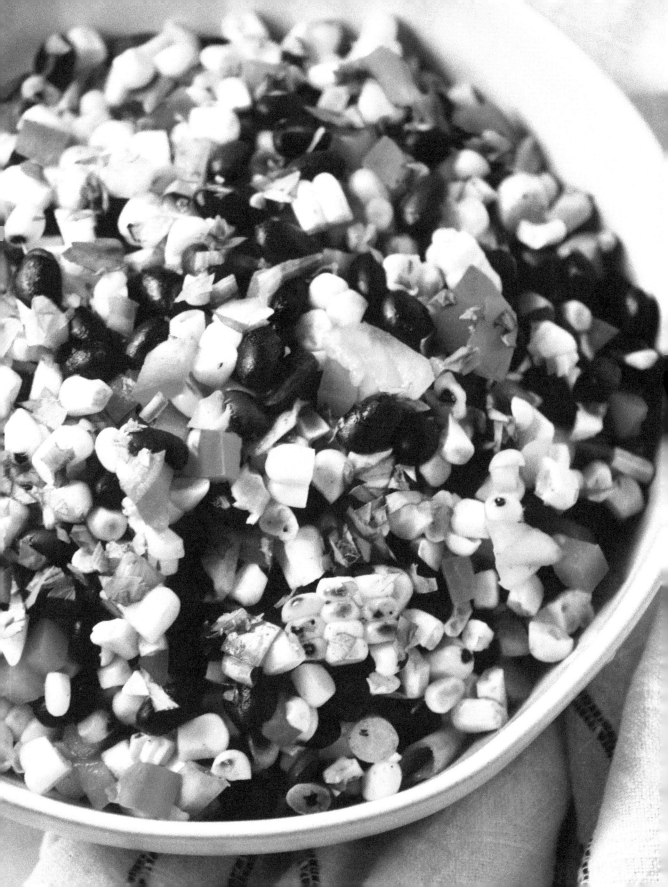

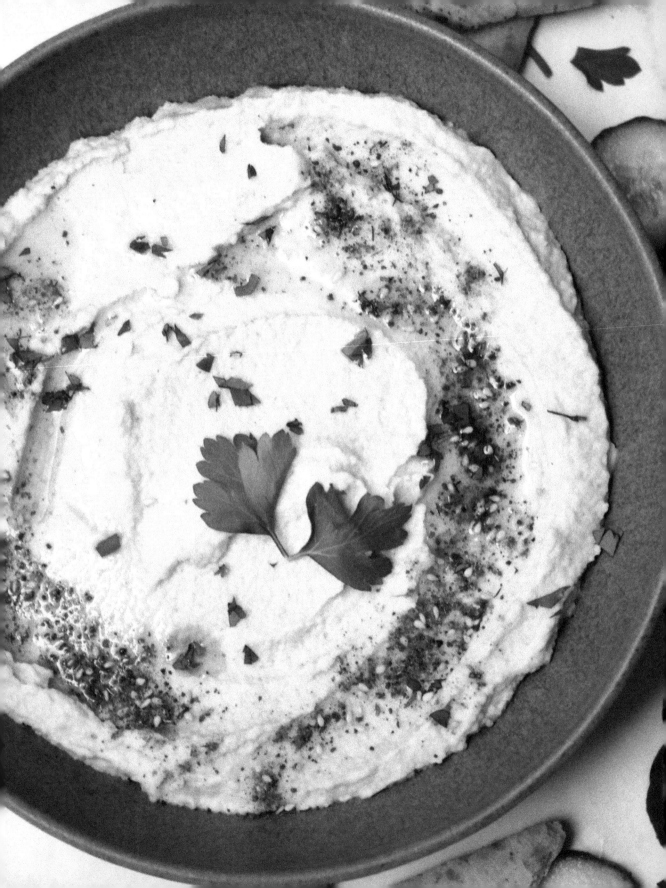

Artichoke Hummus

MAKES ABOUT 1¾ CUPS

Inspired by one of my favorite Greek restaurants in Dallas, this recipe is my favorite way to make hummus. The artichokes give it a great tangy flavor. Use it as a spread on sandwiches, or as a dip paired with pita and vegetables. For the best texture, you'll need a quality, high-powered food processor to break up the fine threads in the artichoke hearts. If you find the texture to be stringy, either the stem or the choke was left on the hearts, or the food processor is not powerful enough.

Half a 14-ounce can garbanzo beans (chickpeas), drained

One 14-ounce can artichoke hearts packed in water, rinsed and drained, excess choke and woody stems trimmed

¼ cup tahini

1 large or 2 small garlic cloves

1 tablespoon distilled white vinegar

½ teaspoon dried oregano

2 tablespoons olive oil

Kosher salt and freshly ground pepper

Za'atar, for sprinkling (optional)

Fresh parsley, chopped or leaves, for serving (optional)

Sliced cucumber, carrots, and celery for dipping

Pita, for serving

Rinse the garbanzo beans in a colander and drain well. Place them on a dish towel and rub them back and forth until dry. Discard the bean skins that fall off.

Put the artichoke hearts in a food processor and chop them. Add the chickpeas, tahini, garlic clove(s), vinegar, and oregano. While blending, slowly add the olive oil until the mixture is emulsified. If you like a thinner consistency, add 1 to 2 tablespoons of cold water to the machine. Season to taste.

Transfer the mixture to a bowl, cover, and refrigerate for at least 30 minutes to let the flavors combine. Top with za'atar and parsley, if desired, and serve with sliced vegetables and pita.

Creamy White Bean & Kale Soup

MAKES 4 TO 6 SERVINGS

The inspiration for this recipe came from the beloved classic, Zuppa Toscana. I wanted all those flavors, but I keep it vegetarian and use white kidney beans, also known as cannellini beans. This is one soup that's amazing the next day, after the spices have had time to really infuse the broth.

1 tablespoon extra-virgin olive oil

2 shallots, chopped

¾ cup chopped or grated carrots

3 garlic cloves, minced

One 15-ounce can cannellini (white kidney) beans, rinsed and drained

1 teaspoon dried oregano

½ teaspoon fennel seeds

¼ teaspoon dried red pepper flakes

4 cups vegetable broth

1 teaspoon kosher salt

2 cups kale, chopped

¼ cup heavy cream

In a large pot, warm the olive oil over medium-high heat. Add the shallots and carrots and sauté until the shallots have softened, about 3 minutes. Reduce the heat to medium and add the garlic, stirring until fragrant, about 1 minute. Mix in the cannellini beans, oregano, fennel, and red pepper flakes and stir until well mixed.

Pour in the broth and salt. Increase the heat to high and bring the liquid to a boil, stirring occasionally. Once boiling, turn down the heat to low to maintain a steady simmer. Stir in the kale and cream and cook until the vegetables are softened, 10 to 15 minutes. Taste and adjust any seasonings.

Divide the soup among serving bowls and serve hot.

NOTE: For a dairy-free, plant-based soup, use unsweetened canned coconut cream instead of heavy cream.

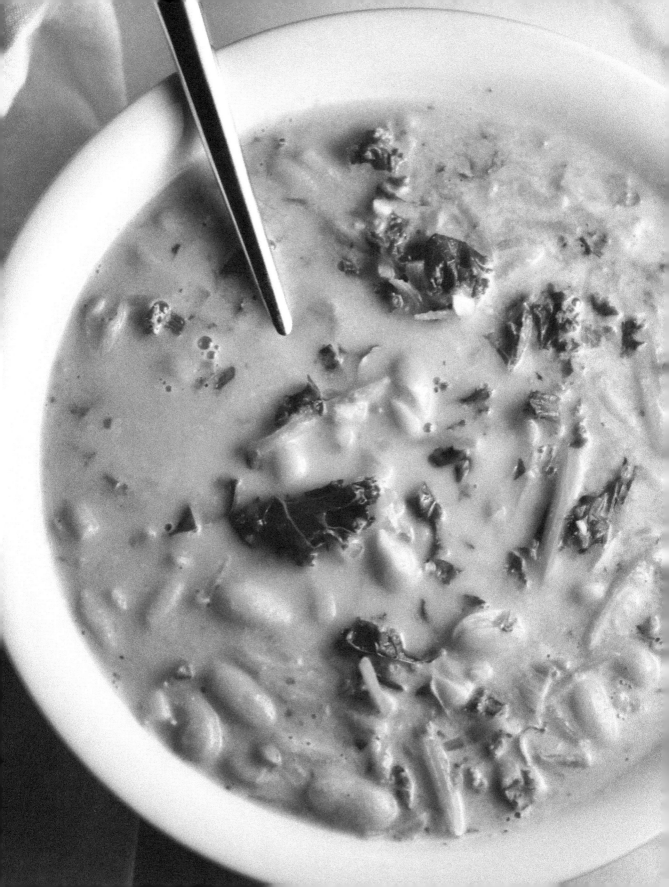

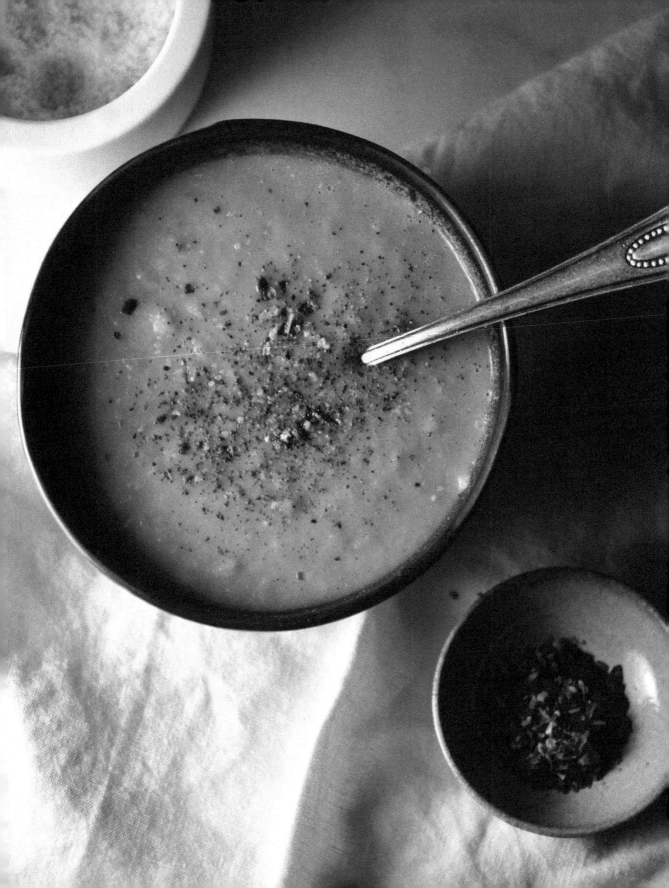

Hearty Lentil Soup

MAKES 6 SERVINGS

Red lentils have a mild, earthy flavor making them perfect for soups and stews. Combined with anti-inflammatory turmeric and lots of vegetables, this is a hearty vegetarian soup that freezes well for up to six months. Although blending it requires one extra step, the texture becomes creamy and thick without using heavy cream.

2 tablespoons extra-virgin olive oil

⅔ cup chopped shallots (about 2 small)

1½ cups chopped carrots

½ cup chopped celery (about 1 large stalk)

2 garlic cloves, minced

2 teaspoons paprika

1½ teaspoons ground cumin

½ teaspoon smoked paprika

½ teaspoon ground turmeric

2 bay leaves

1¾ cups dried red lentils

8 cups vegetable broth

1 tablespoon distilled white vinegar or lemon juice

Kosher salt and freshly ground black pepper

In a large pot, warm the olive oil over medium heat. Add the shallots, carrots, and celery, and sauté until softened, about 3 minutes. Stir in the garlic cloves and cook until fragrant, about 1 minute. Add the paprika, cumin, smoked paprika, turmeric, and bay leaves to the pot and stir until blended. Add the lentils and broth and bring to a simmer over medium-high heat. Reduce the heat to low and simmer gently until the lentils are soft, 25 to 30 minutes.

Remove the bay leaves (very important!). Use an immersion blender to blend the soup until almost smooth; some texture can remain. Alternatively, in batches if necessary, carefully transfer the soup to a full-size blender and blend until smooth. Stir in the vinegar or lemon juice and season with salt and pepper to taste.

Divide the soup among serving bowls and serve warm.

Easy Air-Fried Falafels

MAKES 12 FALAFELS

This version of the Middle Eastern chickpea fritters is super-flavorful, featuring lots of herbs and spices. Topped with a creamy tahini sauce, they make a great vegetarian dinner or snack. These can be fried in a pan, but air frying decreases the amount of oil absorbed making it healthier overall. Be sure to follow the manufacturer's instructions on your air fryer and adjust the cooking time as needed.

TAHINI SAUCE

2 tablespoons tahini

1 garlic clove, minced

1 teaspoon honey

2 teaspoons distilled white vinegar or lemon juice

¼ cup warm water

FALAFELS

One 15-ounce can garbanzo beans, rinsed and drained

½ cup fresh parsley leaves

3 cloves garlic

⅓ cup chopped shallots

1½ teaspoons ground cumin

¾ teaspoon ground coriander

⅓ cup all-purpose flour

Kosher salt and freshly ground black pepper

Olive oil spray

¼ cup toasted sesame seeds

To make the sauce, in a bowl, mix together the tahini, garlic, honey, vinegar, and water until smooth. Set aside.

To make the falafels, rinse the garbanzo beans in a colander and drain well. Place them on a dish towel and rub them back and forth until dry. Discard the bean skins that fall off (it's okay if a few skins remain).

In a food processor, combine the parsley, garlic, shallots, cumin, and coriander. Add the garbanzo beans and pulse quickly just until the mixture is crumbly, about 5 times. Add the flour and pulse another 3 to 4 times to blend. Taste and add salt and pepper as needed—remember as the mixture chills, the flavors will intensify. Transfer the falafel mixture to a freezer-proof bowl and chill in the freezer until cold, about 20 minutes.

Spray the air fryer with olive oil and heat it to 375°F. Use a tablespoon to scoop up the falafel mixture and roll in your hands to form a ball. Press down lightly on the top of the ball to flatten it into a large puck and set aside. Repeat to shape the rest of the mixture. Sprinkle the pucks with sesame seeds.

Place the falafel pucks in the preheated air fryer, at least ½ inch apart. Following the manufacturer's instructions, air-fry the falafels, flipping them halfway, until firm and crispy on the outside with a golden brown hue, 10 to 15 minutes. Air fryers can vary in how fast they cook different foods. Be sure to keep a close eye on the falafel as it cooks. (Alternatively, to fry these in a pan, heat ¼ inch of olive oil in a cast iron skillet over medium-high heat. Add the falafel pucks, and fry until cooked through and brown and crispy on the outside, 2 to 3 minutes per side. Remove with tongs and drain on a paper towel.)

To serve, divide the falafels among plates and drizzle with tahini sauce or place the sauce in a separate bowl for dipping.

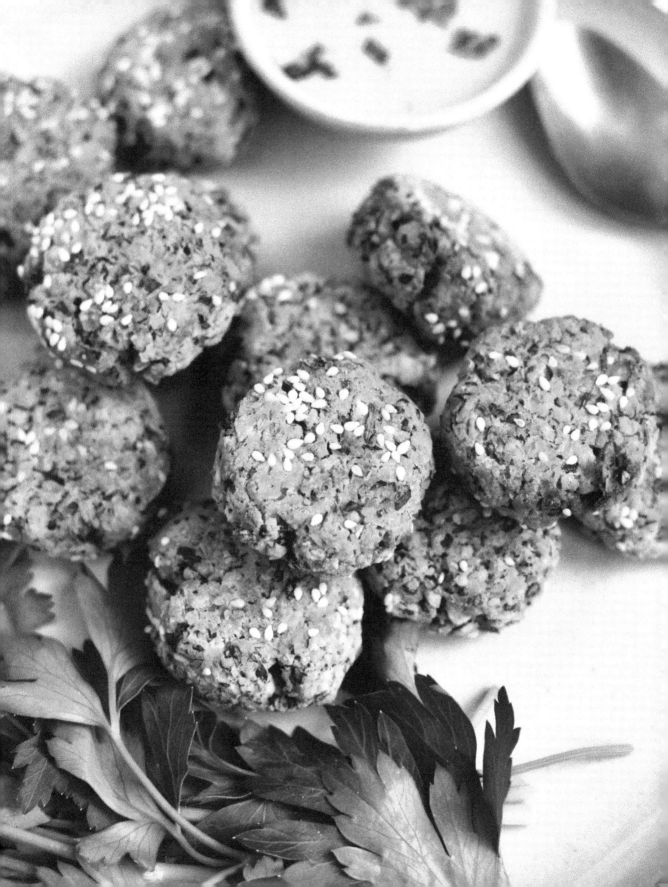

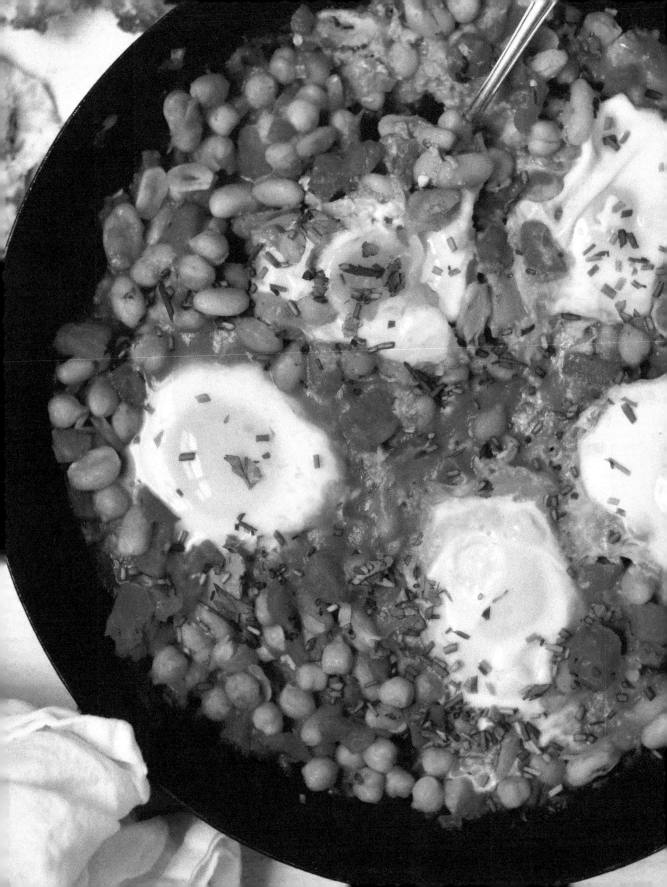

Spanish Bean & Egg Skillet

SERVES 4

Beans and eggs? Yes, it actually works! This quick breakfast, lunch, or dinner is a beautiful dish that pairs perfectly with crusty, warm bread for dipping. If tomatoes are a personal trigger, this is a great time to use the Nomato Sauce (page 96) instead of the canned tomatoes in an equal amount. This pairs well with a mixed green salad and my Basil Vinaigrette (page 79).

1½ tablespoons olive oil

1 large shallot, chopped

4 cloves garlic, minced

1 can (14.5 ounces) diced tomatoes

¾ cup vegetable broth

1 cup canned, rinsed and drained garbanzo beans

1 cup canned, rinsed and drained cannellini beans

1 teaspoon smoked paprika

¾ teaspoon kosher salt

4 to 5 large eggs

1 tablespoon chopped fresh chives

1 tablespoon chopped fresh parsley

Freshly ground black pepper

Warm bread or pita for dipping

Preheat the oven to 375°F. In a large cast-iron pan over medium heat, warm the olive oil. Add the shallot and garlic and sauté until soft, 1 to 2 minutes. Add the tomatoes, broth, garbanzo and cannellini beans, smoked paprika, and salt. Stir to mix the ingredients well. Increase the heat to medium-high and bring to a simmer for about 5 minutes.

Use a wooden spoon to make 4 or 5 little wells in the bean mixture. Carefully crack each egg and gently slide them into the wells, keeping the egg intact. Transfer the pan to the oven and bake, until the egg whites have set but the yolks still jiggle, 10 to 13 minutes for runny yolks, or until cooked to your liking. Remove from the oven and top with chives, parsley and pepper to taste.

To serve, use a large spoon to divide the bean mixture and eggs among serving plates. Serve as is or with crusty, warm bread or pita for dipping.

Chickpea Mayonnaise

MAKES ABOUT 1 CUP

This easy mayonnaise recipe uses chickpeas and their liquid (aquafaba) instead of eggs for a fluffy and creamy spread. Use an immersion blender, and follow the directions carefully for the best results. You can also use a good-quality food processor for this, but I find the immersion blender to be more foolproof for beginners. The mixture is more like an aioli when first made and at room temperature; it will thicken to a traditional mayo-like consistency as it cools in the refrigerator.

1 tablespoon distilled white vinegar

½ teaspoon mustard powder

3 tablespoons aquafaba, drained from a can of chickpeas

12 whole chickpeas from the can

½ teaspoon kosher salt, or to taste

½ cup plus 1 tablespoon avocado oil

2 tablespoons olive oil

Pinch of sugar, if needed

In the tall cup that comes with the immersion blender, combine the vinegar, mustard powder, aquafaba, chickpeas, and salt. Blend until smooth and frothy.

With the blender on high, drizzle in the oils VERY slowly, pausing when needed to allow the mixture to become thick and creamy. If you add the oil too fast, you'll end up with an oily mess. Continue blending until the texture is more like a thick aioli rather than a dressing. The whole process takes 1 to 2 minutes. Once it reaches that thickness, stop blending immediately.

Taste and adjust the seasonings, adding a pinch of sugar if it's tart or bitter. Store in the refrigerator in a mason jar or airtight container for up to 2 weeks.

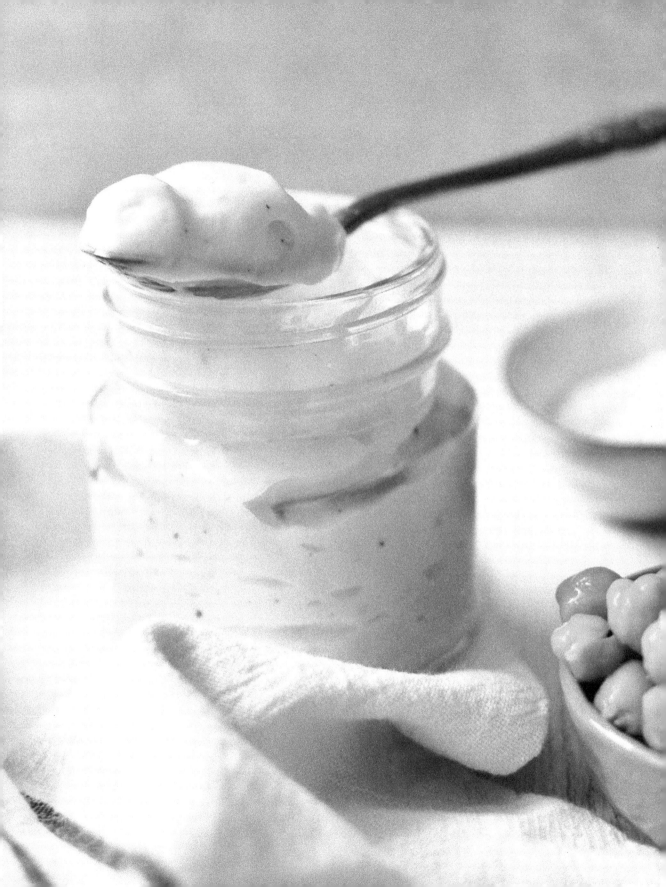

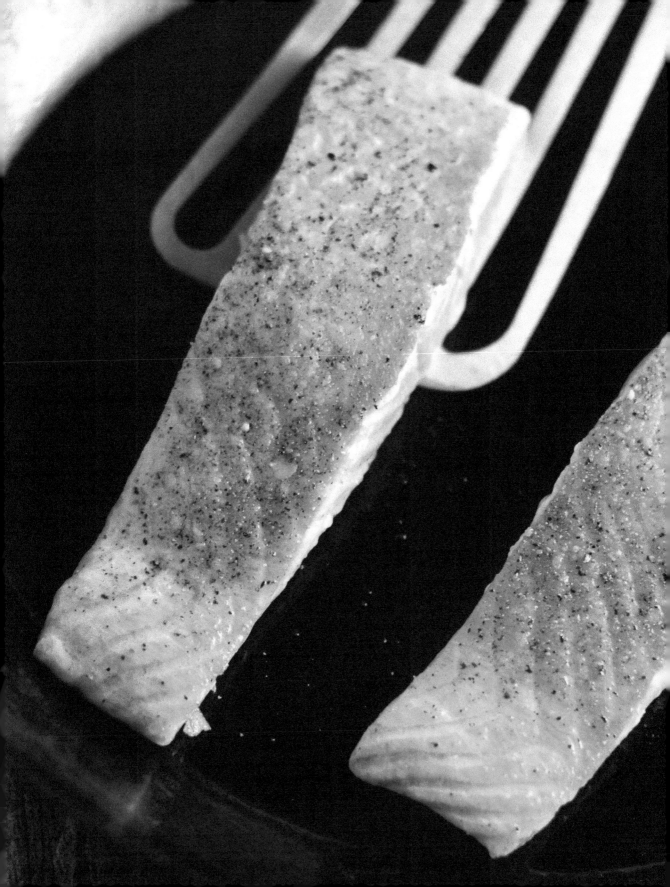

FISH & SHELLFISH

THE BENEFITS OF FISH & SHELLFISH

Because the Mediterranean region surrounds a sea, seafood forms the primary protein source and is consumed on an almost daily basis. Fish (particularly fatty fish like salmon, trout, cod, herring, and halibut), marine crustaceans (e.g., shrimp, lobster, and crab), and marine mollusks (e.g., squids, octopuses, clams, and mussels) are a great source of omega-3 fatty acids, coenzyme-Q10, vitamin D, magnesium, copper, zinc, niacin, selenium, and carotenoids (astraxanthin and fucoxanthin). Omega-3 fatty acids and nutrients from seafood have numerous health benefits, including for brain health. In fact, omega-3 fatty acids may have played a huge role in human evolution. According to archaeologist Curtis Marean, approximately 200,000 years ago, our ancestors began foraging on shellfish, and the big dietary increase in omega-3 fatty acid and marine nutrients helped promote human brain evolution.

Unfortunately, due to pollution, marine life has been contaminated with heavy metals. Larger and longer-living fish like tuna, swordfish, marlin, and king mackerel consume smaller fish, and thus accumulate higher levels of mercury. Mercury is a neurotoxin that can be harmful. Crustaceans and mollusks may be contaminated with cadmium, another potentially toxic heavy metal. In general, according to the FDA, adults should limit intake of low-mercury seafood to 3 to 5 ounces twice per week to limit heavy metal exposure. Women who are pregnant or breastfeeding should consult with their doctors for advice on eating fish and shellfish.

SHOPPING FOR FISH & SHELLFISH

To some cooks, preparing seafood can be intimidating. I'm hoping my tips give a little bit of confidence to show how easy it is to incorporate this amazing brain food into your diet.

When choosing shellfish or fish, it's important to have a nice chat with the fishmonger. First, you'll want to know when the fish was received in the shop. Next, judge for yourself how fresh it seems. A good way to tell if a fillet or steak is fresh is to ask the fishmonger if you can give your selection a quick smell. It shouldn't smell "fishy," rather, ocean fish should smell like seawater and freshwater fish should smell like a lake or stream. If it seems pungent, you may want to pass.

Ask for "dry scallops," which are not injected with phosphates to plump them up and add weight. Dry scallops look more cream or tan colored, versus wet scallops which are greyish or very white. Because they're not water-logged, dry scallops sear really well and also have a sweet, buttery flavor to them.

Numbers next to shrimp, like U-15 and 21/25, indicate how many shrimp are typically in a pound based on sizing. The recipes here will work for any type or size of shrimp you enjoy, so pick what is available or what you prefer. The most important thing is that they are peeled and deveined, which most stores carry now. A lot of frozen shrimp are packed with sodium tripolyphosphate, similar to scallops. It's worth the search to find some without it from both a taste and migraine standpoint.

With crab, I recommend jumbo lump for crab cakes, which usually is packed in a small container and refrigerated in stores. Buying crab meat fresh instead of canned yields a better flavor and texture overall when it comes to crab cakes. However, if you're just adding crab to a salad, a good quality canned will work! The same goes for canned fish. Look for tuna and salmon packed in oil or water, with no broths, solutions, or flavorings.

When buying a whole fish, like a branzino, look at the eyes: They should be clear and not cloudy. Then, peer at the gills: They should be bright red and not brown. Another tip when buying a whole fish is to ask the fishmonger to clean it and prep it for you. They will check for errant scales and cut it any way you want.

If the fish is already wrapped in plastic, look for a package without excess water inside.

And if purchasing frozen fish, grab a bag that's near the coldest part of the freezer with a recent packed on date. It's best to thaw the fish overnight in the refrigerator; for a quick thawing method, put the sealed package in a bowl of cold water for 30 to 60 minutes.

From a health perspective, many types of wild-caught fish can be better choices than farmed fish; that said, I actually prefer the milder flavor of farmed salmon over the stronger flavor of wild. If this your preference, too, look for sustainably farmed and ocean-safe options like Verlasso salmon, which try to mimic what the fish would eat in the wild for a similar omega-3 content. While there can be a wide variance in omega-3 content when comparing farmed fish to wild (wild tends to have less fat and therefore less omega-3s, but also less saturated fat), the difference shouldn't be enough to greatly affect your purchasing decisions, especially since wild can be so much more expensive.

When purchasing fresh clams or mussels, look for whole shells that are not cracked and are completely closed. Ask the fishmonger to discard any cracked ones or to tap ones that are slightly open. When tapped, the clam or mussel should close shut, indicating if it's still alive. It's very important to keep clams and mussels alive until cooking. I recommend always purchasing them the day you plan to cook them and storing them the refrigerator or on ice with the bag open so that they can "breathe."

If you live in an area with limited access to good, fresh fish and shellfish, consider investing in a seafood delivery service like Fish Fixe. I find the quality is typically very good and I like the pre-portioned options. It's the next best thing to having a really good fishmonger in your neighborhood.

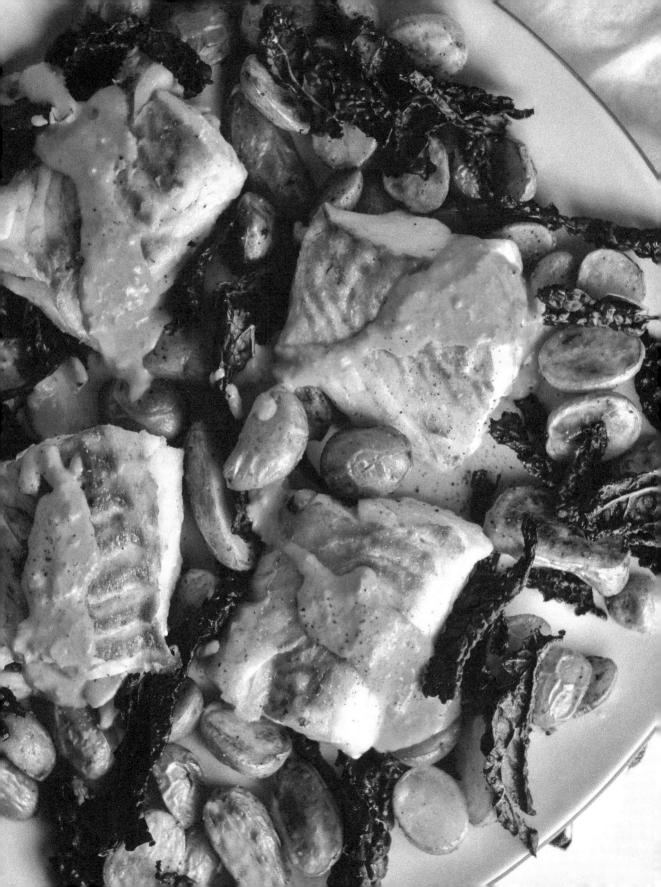

Patatas Bravas with Cod & Crispy Kale

MAKES 4 SERVINGS AND ABOUT 1 CUP OF SAUCE

Spain was my first international destination after being diagnosed with vestibular migraine, and although I didn't always navigate the amazing hot chocolate and jamon iberico without an attack, I did my best to immerse myself in the culture and food despite living with a migraine disorder. Siestas were helpful! One of my favorite tapas was patatas bravas, which are crispy fried potatoes with a spicy, smoky sauce and garlic aioli. This version is definitely not traditional, but it combines all the great flavors into a creamy bravas-style sauce that pairs well with the fish and crispy kale. This preparation would also work with halibut, trout, or branzino, but watch the cooking time on the fish if you have thin fillets. If you have leftover sauce, it pairs well with the Tart Cherry Grilled Steak (page 215) and roasted potatoes prepared with these instructions.

1¼ pounds fingerling or baby yellow potatoes, sliced in half

Extra-virgin olive oil or olive oil spray

7 ounces lacinato kale, washed and spun dry, thick stems removed, torn into large pieces

Kosher salt and freshly ground black pepper

Preheat the oven to 425°F. Line a large, rimmed baking sheet with parchment paper.

Put the potatoes on the prepared baking sheet. Drizzle with 2 teaspoons olive oil (or spray generously) and a pinch of kosher salt and pepper and toss well. Roast, flipping the potatoes halfway, until golden brown and crispy, 20 to 25 minutes. Remove from the oven and turn the oven heat down to 375°F.

Transfer the potatoes to a serving platter and place the kale on the same baking sheet. Toss the kale with 2 teaspoons olive oil, rubbing it with your fingers, and sprinkle lightly with salt and pepper. Bake until dried out and crispy (they will crisp up more as they cool), 6 to 9 minutes. Smaller pieces of kale may burn before the rest is ready, so pull them out of the oven if they are starting to turn black. Remove the kale from the oven and transfer to the serving platter along with the potatoes.

BRAVAS SAUCE

2 tablespoons extra-virgin olive oil

1 small shallot, chopped

2 garlic cloves, minced

2 teaspoons Spanish sweet smoked paprika

¼ to ½ teaspoon hot smoked paprika

1 Roma tomato, seeds and pulp removed, roughly chopped

½ cup mayonnaise

1 teaspoon distilled white vinegar

Kosher salt and freshly ground black pepper to taste

Four 4- to 6-ounce cod fillets, skin removed

To make the bravas sauce, in a nonstick skillet over medium heat, warm the 2 tablespoons olive oil. Add the shallot and garlic and cook, stirring often with a wooden spoon, until softened and fragrant, 1 to 2 minutes. Add the sweet and hot smoked paprika, stirring for about 1 minute to warm the spices. Transfer the mixture to a food processor. Add the chopped tomato, mayonnaise, and vinegar and process until smooth. Taste, adding salt and pepper as needed. Set aside.

Wipe out the same pan and place over medium-high heat. Add 1 tablespoon olive oil. Once hot, add the cod fillets, placing them down on the side where the skin used to be (it will be darker). Let the fish sear, without touching, for 5 minutes; it should be golden brown. Carefully flip the fish and cook until golden brown on the other side and the center is no longer translucent, another 4 to 5 minutes.

To serve, arrange the cod fillets on the serving platter with the potatoes and kale. Top with the bravas sauce or place the sauce in a dish on the side for dipping. The bravas sauce will keep covered in an airtight container in the refrigerator for up to 1 week.

TIP: A note on paprika—Spanish sweet smoked paprika balances hot smoked paprika, and it's worth the investment to try to find them both for this sauce. It is not the same flavor as regular smoked paprika that is available at most grocery stores, which will work in a pinch, but won't be quite as good. I found both at my local Central Market, but they are also available online. I recommend starting with ¼ teaspoon of the hot paprika, adding more to the sauce later on if needed. In my opinion, the sauce has just a hint of spiciness without being too hot, but I like to give options!

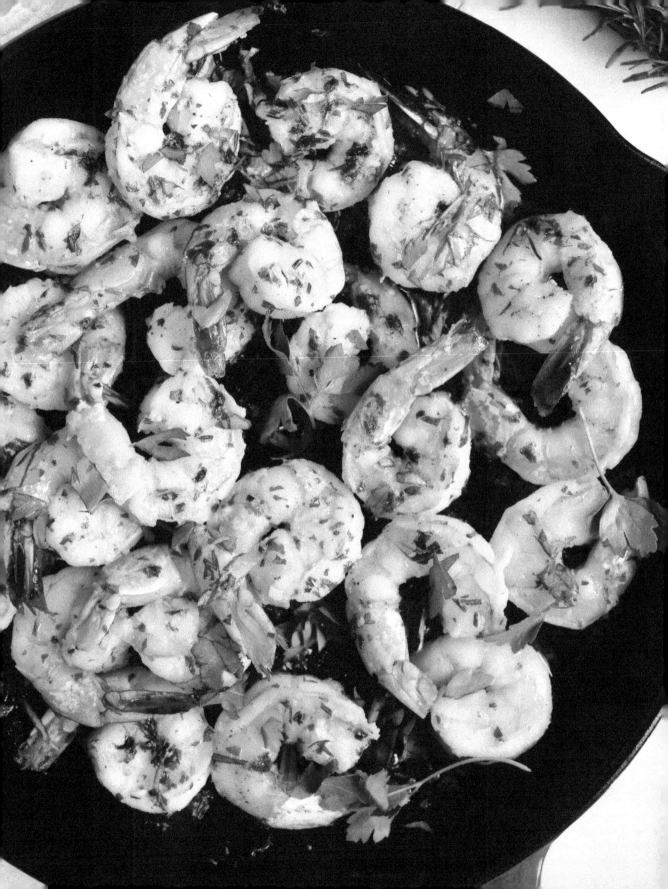

Garlic-Herb Shrimp

MAKES 4 SERVINGS

If you're looking for a quick yet impressive dinner, this one is it. This recipe was inspired by one of my favorite Spanish dishes, gambas al ajillo, which tastes super decadent considering it uses such simple ingredients. Cooking shrimp in a large amount of olive oil gives it such a luscious flavor, but a mixture of fresh herbs cuts the richness and provides a light counterpart to the dish. If you tolerate citrus well, you can set out lemon wedges at serving time.

½ cup extra-virgin olive oil

4 garlic cloves

1 tablespoon chopped fresh rosemary

¾ cup fresh parsley leaves

1 tablespoon distilled white vinegar or lemon juice

1½ pounds peeled and deveined shrimp, tail-on optional (16 to 25 size recommended)

Kosher salt and black pepper

In a small food processor, combine the olive oil, garlic, rosemary, ½ cup of the parsley, and the vinegar or lemon juice. Turn on the machine and process until relatively smooth (some larger pieces of parsley can remain). Transfer to a shallow dish.

Add the shrimp to the herb mixture and toss well. If you have time, place the shrimp in the refrigerator to marinate for 30 minutes.

Place a large nonstick or cast-iron pan over medium to medium-high heat. Carefully add the shrimp and marinade to the pan and cook, stirring occasionally with a wooden spoon, until the shrimp are opaque, 2 to 3 minutes.

Transfer the shrimp to a serving platter and season to taste with salt and pepper. Sprinkle with the remaining ¼ cup parsley and serve right away.

Seared Scallops with Vegetable Ragout

MAKES 4 SERVINGS

Don't be intimidated by scallops! I give you all the tips you need here for the perfect sear. Start with really good scallops that haven't been injected with phosphates to plump them up—these are called "dry" scallops. They're typically a milky, creamy color and not stark white or grey. They're also more expensive than treated scallops because they're large without added water weight. The best part is that they sear beautifully. Good quality, dry white wines are generally better tolerated for people with migraine. If you are sensitive to sulfites, I recommend either using a PureWine Wine Wand before adding the wine to the pan or substituting broth. While cooking dramatically reduces the alcohol in a dish, it unfortunately doesn't eliminate sulfites in wine. For those sensitive to citrus, use sumac, which has a great tangy flavor.

1½ pounds dry sea scallops (see note above)

1 tablespoon extra-virgin olive oil

¼ cup vegetable broth or white wine

½ cup chopped shallots

4 ears corn (about 2 cups of kernels)

1 cup chopped red bell pepper

1 cup green beans, trimmed and chopped

2 large garlic cloves, minced

Finely grated zest of 1 lemon, or 1 teaspoon sumac

3 cups fresh spinach leaves

½ teaspoon kosher salt

Freshly ground black pepper

Pat dry the scallops and place them on a plate. Set them in the refrigerator for 15 to 20 minutes (this helps them dry out more for a nice sear).

Warm a large nonstick or cast-iron skillet over medium-high heat and add the olive oil. Season the scallops with fresh pepper (I find they're already salty, so I do not use salt). Arrange the scallops in the pan at least 1 to 2 inches apart. Now, don't touch them! Let them sear until golden on the bottom and you can easily pull them off the bottom of the pan, about 2 minutes. If you turn the scallops too early, they can stick to the pan. Using tongs, turn them to the other side and cook until just golden brown and cooked through, about 2 more minutes. Do not overcook the scallops or they turn rubbery. Transfer the seared scallops to a plate, cover with foil, and keep warm.

Reduce the heat under the pan to medium and carefully pour the broth or wine into the hot pan, scraping up any browned bits with a wooden spoon. Add the shallots, corn kernels, bell pepper, and green beans, stirring frequently, until the vegetables are softened, 4 to 5 minutes. Add the garlic and lemon zest or sumac. Stir and cook for another 2 minutes to blend the flavors. Add the spinach and cook until wilted, 30 to 60 seconds. Season with kosher salt and pepper to taste.

To serve, divide the vegetable mixture among serving plates and place the seared scallops on top. Serve right away.

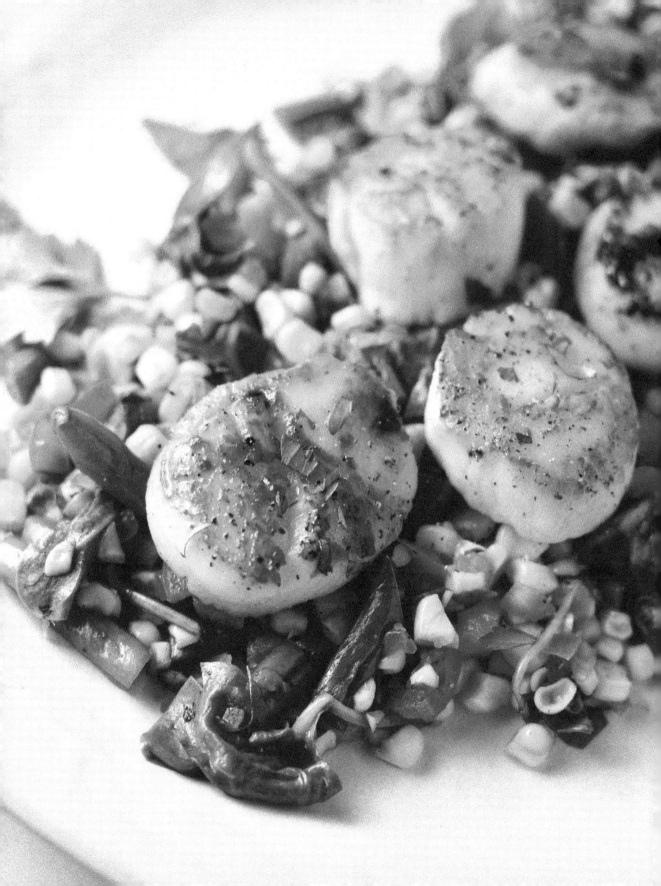

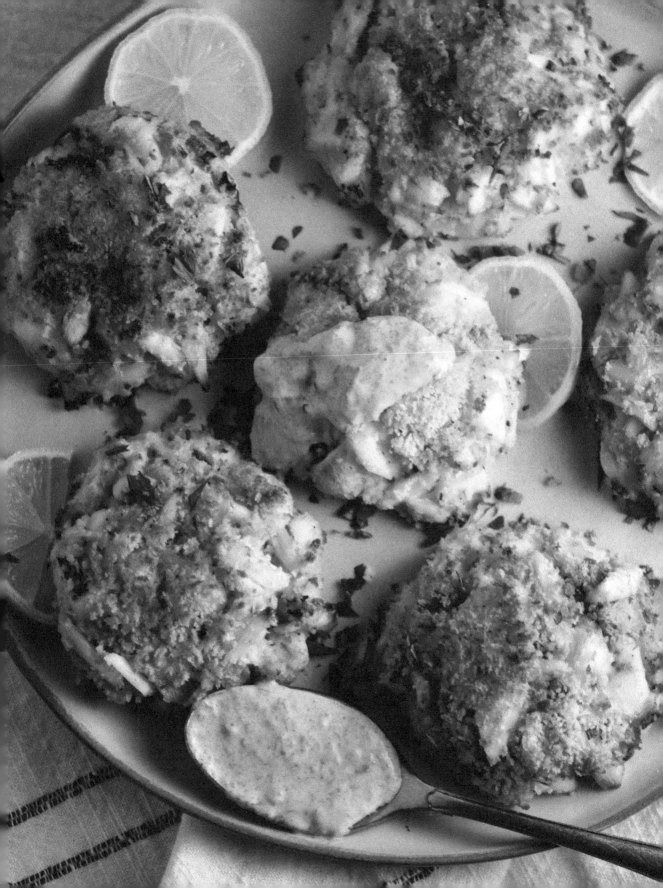

Baked Crab Cakes with Red Pepper Aioli

MAKES 6

Here is a healthier take on crab cakes that are baked instead of fried and topped with a roasted red pepper aioli. You can simply buy roasted red peppers, but they're easy to make at home: Spray them with olive oil and roast in a 500°F oven until black spots form on the outside of the skin, about 10 minutes per side. I roast the peppers ahead and store them in a Mason jar for up to 1 week.

ROASTED RED PEPPER AIOLI
¼ cup roasted red peppers
⅓ cup mayonnaise
¼ teaspoon smoked paprika

CRAB CAKES
¼ cup mayonnaise
½ teaspoon paprika
½ teaspoon celery seed
1 large egg, whisked
1 tablespoon Dijon mustard
¼ cup chopped green onion
¾ cup panko
16 ounces fresh jumbo lump crab, picked free of any shell pieces

To make the aioli, in a food processor, combine the roasted red peppers, mayonnaise, and smoked paprika. Blend until smooth. Transfer to a bowl and refrigerate until ready to use.

To make the crab cakes, in a large bowl, combine the mayonnaise, paprika and celery seed, egg, mustard, green onion, and ½ cup of the panko. Mix until blended, then gently stir in the lump crab meat with a rubber spatula, being careful to not break it apart. Chill the mixture for 30 to 60 minutes. The longer it chills, the easier it will be to form.

Preheat the oven to 450°F. Line a rimmed baking sheet with parchment paper.

Form the crab mixture into 6 equal mounds. Press the remaining ¼ cup panko on the tops and bake until firm and golden brown on the outside, about 15 minutes. If not already light brown on top, turn the broiler to high and broil until light brown, about 1 extra minute.

Serve warm with red pepper aioli on the side.

NOTE: For gluten-free crabcakes, use gluten-free panko.

TIP: A lot of store-bought mayonnaise contains oils that are high in omega-6 like soybean, which are best balanced by consuming omega-3s. Although you have a lot of balance in this recipe with omega-3-rich crab, using a homemade or store-bought mayonnaise prepared with olive oil or avocado oil can help make this recipe more brain-healthy. See page 134 for a plant-based avocado oil mayonnaise made from chickpeas.

Steamed Clams with Fresh Herbs

MAKES 2 MAIN-DISH OR 4 SIDE-DISH SERVINGS

This recipe uses littleneck clams, but mussels work well, too, and are also high in omega-3s. If you're using mussels, remove the fibrous "beard" from each shell by yanking it toward the back of the shell. The simple herbed broth highlights the natural briny flavor in the shellfish. Pair it with crusty bread and a bright green salad, like the Asparagus and Pea Salad (page 79).

2 pounds littleneck clams
2 tablespoons olive oil
1 shallot, chopped
3 garlic cloves, minced
1 cup vegetable broth
½ cup fresh parsley leaves, roughly chopped
3 tablespoons chives, minced
Freshly ground black pepper
Warm crusty bread for serving

Fill a large bowl with ice water. Using a stiff-bristled brush, scrub the clams under running water, then place them into the bowl of ice water. Discard any clams that don't close when lightly tapped on the counter or have a crack in the shell. Let the clams soak in the ice water for 20 minutes to remove any sand and grit.

Carefully pull out the clams one by one (don't pour the water out or the grit and sand will go back over them) and place them on a towel.

In a large Dutch oven or heavy-duty pot with a lid, warm the olive oil over medium heat. Add the shallot and garlic and cook, stirring with a wooden spoon, until softened and fragrant, 1 to 2 minutes. Add the broth and clams. Bring the liquid to a simmer and cover with the lid. Cook until all the clams have opened, 6 to 7 minutes. (Sometimes it helps to poke the stubborn ones with a wooden spoon to get them to open. If they haven't opened after a few more minutes, discard them.)

Toss in the parsley, chives, and black pepper to taste. To serve this family-style, using a large spoon, carefully transfer the clams to a serving bowl to prevent breaking the shells and pour the sauce over the top. Or spoon into small bowls if offering personal portions. Serve with warm crusty bread for dipping in the herb broth.

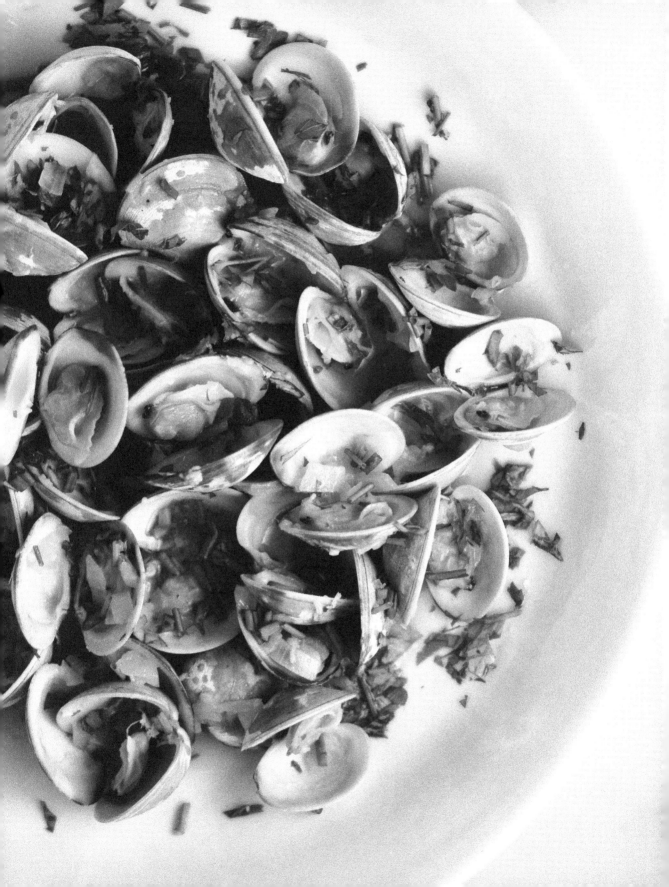

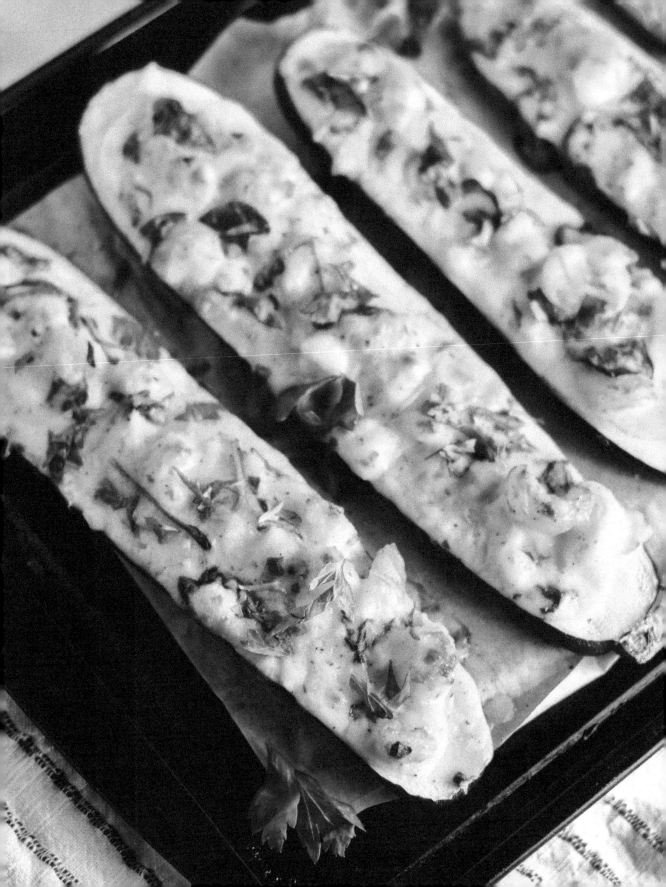

Shrimp Alfredo Zucchini Boats

MAKES 6 LARGE OR 12 SMALL ZUCCHINI BOATS

My favorite alfredo sauce knockoff, which doesn't contain aged cheese, is my
Boursin Pasta—one of the most popular recipes I've ever created. It's creamy and flavorful
without the addition of tyramine-rich Parmesan. This recipe uses that same sauce but
it's mixed with shrimp in a low carb—and more veggies!—way, stuffed in zucchini boats.
This recipe was a suggestion from Dr. Beh, so if you like it, don't forget to thank him!

---

3 large zucchini (about ½ pound each) or 6 to 7 smaller zucchini (about ¼ pound each)

2 teaspoons olive oil, plus more for coating the zucchini

Kosher salt and freshly ground black pepper

2 garlic cloves, minced

2 tablespoons all-purpose flour

½ cup broth

1 cup milk

1 pound shrimp, peeled, deveined, and chopped

3 ounces (half of a 6-ounce package) Boursin Garlic and Fine Herbs cheese

2 cups fresh spinach, roughly chopped

2 tablespoons chopped fresh parsley

Preheat the oven to 425°F. Line a large baking sheet with parchment paper and set aside.

Cut the zucchini in half lengthwise. Using a kitchen spoon, run it down the length of each zucchini half to scoop out the centers to form narrow "boats." Save the scooped zucchini to add to smoothies or the Artichoke Hummus (page 125) to sneak in some extra vegetables. Set the zucchini boats on the prepared baking sheet. If their bottoms are too round and they tend to roll, use a knife to thinly shave off the roundest part, without cutting through to the boat. This will help them lay flat. Lightly drizzle the zucchini boats with olive oil, rubbing all over the inside and outside, then very lightly season them with salt and pepper.

In a large frying pan over medium heat, warm the 2 teaspoons olive oil. Add the garlic and sauté until fragrant, about 30 seconds. Add the flour and stir with a wooden spoon until the garlic is well coated. Pour in the broth, which should sizzle on contact, and stir to scrape up any browned bits on the bottom of the pan. Slowly add the milk a little at a time, stirring until smooth after each addition. Add the shrimp and bring to a simmer. Cook, stirring occasionally, until thickened (the sauce should leave a line when you slide the spoon through) and until the shrimp is cooked through, about 8 minutes. Turn off the heat and fold in the cheese and spinach until the cheese is melted. Taste and add salt and pepper to taste.

Spoon the shrimp mixture into the zucchini boats, dividing evenly. Bake until lightly browned on top and bubbly, 20 to 25 minutes. (If using small zucchini, go with a shorter cooking time of 10 to 15 minutes as they should have a slight crunch when serving.) Top with parsley and black pepper. Serve warm.

Open-Face Fish Salad Sandwich

MAKES 4 SERVINGS

This is a recipe I have been making for years and I often enjoy with friends and family on our patio during a warm summer night. Paired with crispy chips and a cool drink, it makes you feel like you're on a beach vacation! Halibut is not native to the Mediterranean, but it is easy to find at a fish market and has just the right texture and mild flavor to star in this recipe. Spoon on top of toasted bread with a little bit of arugula for a refreshing meal. If you are sensitive to sun-dried tomatoes, replace them with chopped roasted red peppers or omit from the recipe.

1½ pounds fresh halibut or other mild, flaky white fish

Olive oil

Kosher salt and freshly ground black pepper

3 tablespoons mayonnaise

2 garlic cloves, minced

1½ tablespoons minced fresh basil

2 teaspoons minced fresh parsley

1 teaspoon capers, washed, drained, and roughly chopped

3 tablespoons sun-dried tomatoes, chopped

2 teaspoons fresh lemon juice (about ½ lemon) or distilled white vinegar

Toasted bread slices for serving (I like ciabatta)

Arugula for serving

Preheat the oven to 425°F and line a rimmed baking sheet with parchment paper.

Pat the halibut dry. Place the fish skin-side down on the prepared baking sheet and lightly coat with olive oil. Sprinkle lightly with salt and pepper. Bake until just cooked through, 15 to 17 minutes.

Let the halibut cool on the pan for 10 to 15 minutes. Peel off and discard the skin. Break the halibut into large chunks.

In a large bowl, mix together the mayonnaise, garlic, basil, parsley, capers, sun-dried tomatoes, fresh lemon juice or vinegar, and ¼ teaspoon freshly cracked pepper. Stir in the halibut chunks. Refrigerate for at least 30 minutes to allow the flavors to meld together.

Meanwhile, toast bread slices in a toaster or place them on a baking sheet, drizzle the top of the bread with a little olive oil, and toast under the broiler on high for about 1 minute or just till golden brown.

When ready to serve, spoon the fish salad on top of bread slices and top with arugula.

The salad will keep for up to 2 days, tightly covered in the refrigerator.

NOTE: For a gluten-free dish, use your favorite gluten-free bread or serve on top of greens.

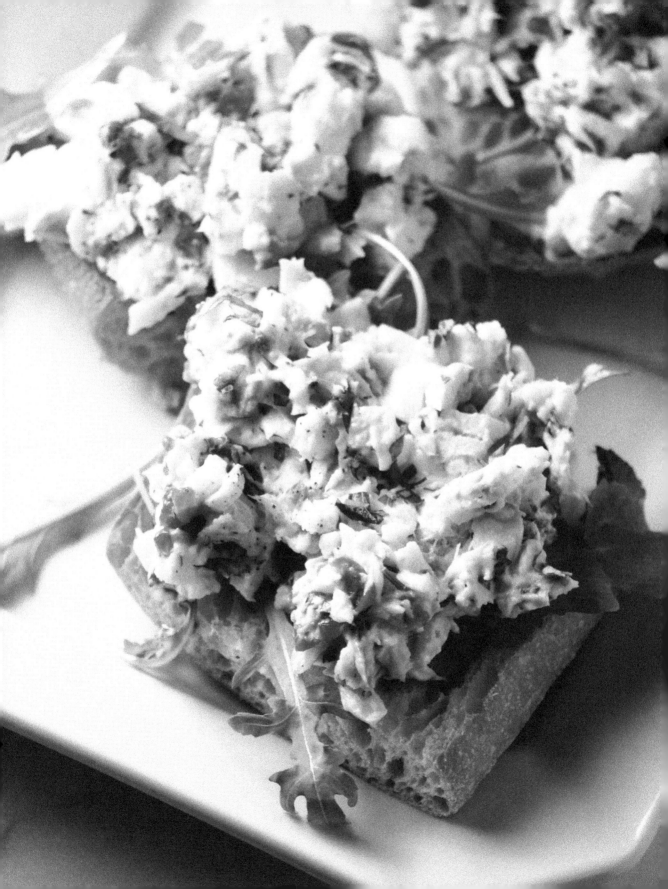

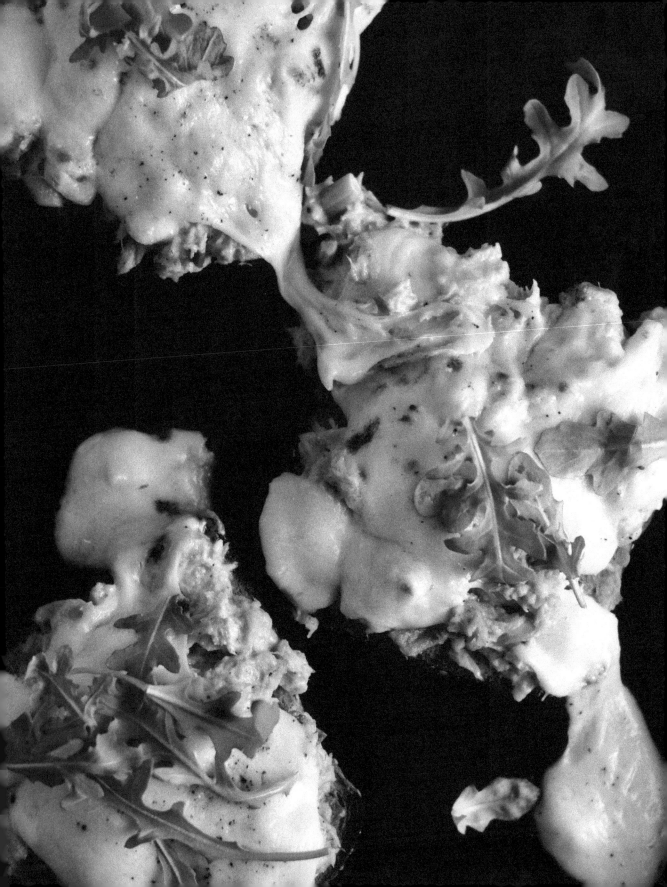

Mozzarella Tuna Melts

MAKES 4 SERVINGS

This recipe was on repeat during my early postpartum days. It's a balanced, nutritious meal with lots of protein, especially when paired with a simple salad. Best of all, it takes less than 10 minutes to make. Tuna melts are usually nothing fancy, but the mustard and olive oil here take it to the next level. Both water-packed and tuna in oil can be used for this recipe, but if using tuna in oil just omit the added olive oil. I recommend Wild Planet or Safe Catch for additive- and sodium-free tuna options. Avoid any brands packed in broth, with flavorings, or with added salt.

4 slices whole-grain bread
Two 5-ounce cans tuna in
    water, no salt added, drained
¼ cup mayonnaise
2 tablespoons sulfite-free
    Dijon mustard
2 small green onions, chopped
2 teaspoons olive oil
Fresh black pepper
4 slices mozzarella cheese
Fresh arugula

Toast the bread until golden brown and set on a baking sheet. Set the broiler to high.

In a bowl, combine the tuna, mayonnaise, mustard, green onions, olive oil, and black pepper to taste. Top the toasted bread slices with the tuna mixture, dividing evenly, then top each with a piece of mozzarella.

Place the baking sheet under the broiler and broil, watching carefully, until the cheese is just melted, 1 to 2 minutes.

Divide the melts among serving plates, top with fresh arugula, and serve slightly warm.

NOTE: For a gluten-free dish, use your favorite gluten-free bread.

Whole Roasted Branzino with Fresh Herbs

MAKES 3 WHOLE FISH (4 SERVINGS TOTAL)

This dinner is delicious, healthy, and impressive, with tons of fresh flavor. I love recipes like this to challenge myself to try new things in the kitchen. Try this for a date night or a small dinner party. If you want a sauce to pair with this dish, I recommend my Red Pepper Aioli (page 151).

1 pound fingerling potatoes, sliced in half

1 tablespoon plus 2 teaspoons olive oil

Kosher salt and freshly ground black pepper

3 whole branzino (Mediterranean sea bass) or red snapper, about 1 pound each, cleaned, rinsed, and patted dry

8 garlic cloves, minced

¼ teaspoon freshly ground black pepper

1 lemon, thinly sliced

6 sprigs fresh rosemary

6 sprigs fresh parsley

Preheat the oven to 400°F. Line a large, rimmed baking sheet with parchment paper.

In a bowl, toss the potatoes with 2 teaspoons of the olive oil. Season lightly with salt and pepper and toss well. Transfer the potatoes to the prepared baking sheet and roast for 10 minutes. Remove from the oven and nudge the potatoes around to make room for the fish.

Increase the oven heat to 450°F. In a bowl, combine the remaining 1 tablespoon olive oil, minced garlic, and ¼ teaspoon pepper. Rub this mixture inside and outside of each fish, avoiding the head and tail. Sprinkle with salt. Stuff the fish cavities with lemon slices and rosemary and parsley sprigs, dividing evenly. Place on the baking sheet with the potatoes and roast until the fish is opaque, not translucent, about 20 minutes. Remove from the oven and let stand for 5 minutes.

To fillet the fish, using two large spoons, break away the head and the tail (they should come away easily) and discard. Remove the lemon and herbs from the cavities and scrape away any extra fins from the bottom of the fish. Run the spoon along the top edge of the fish, removing the bones. Then use the back of a knife to gently slide the flesh off the skin on the side of the fish that is facing you.

Starting at the tail section, slide a knife or a thin pie server in the center of the fish, just resting on top of the bones, and carefully lift to remove the fish fillet. Place that fillet on a serving plate. Removing the fillet will reveal the spine in the center of the fish—lift it out in one piece to get to the other fillet. Gently slide the knife between the skin and the fillet and lift the fillet out, placing it on the serving plate.

Run your fingers carefully along the fillets to check for stray bones. Surround the fillets with fresh herbs, lemon slices, and potatoes.

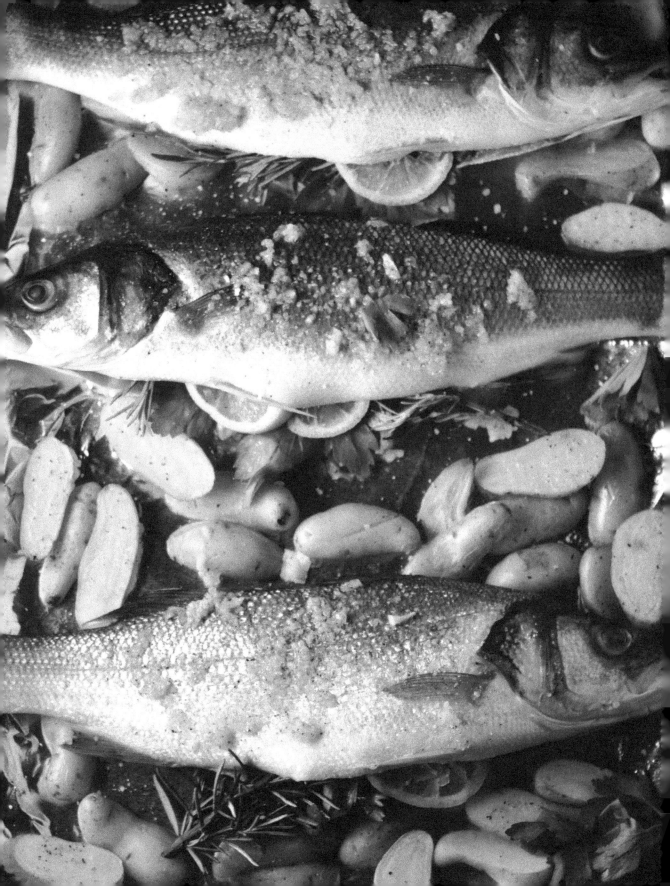

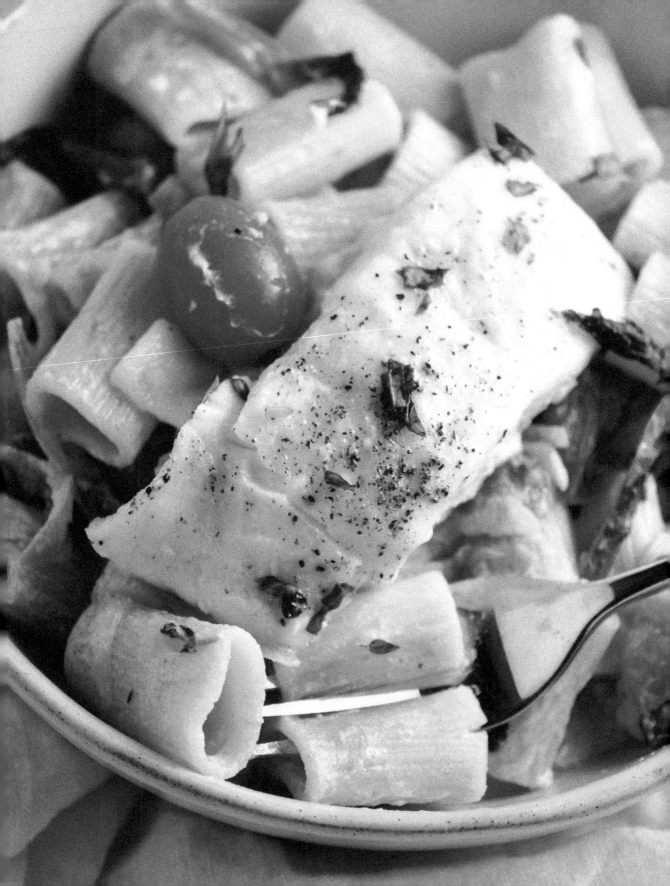

Baked Halibut & Goat Cheese Pasta

MAKES 3 TO 4 SERVINGS

The idea behind this cooking method became famous as "TikTok pasta," made with baked feta. Personally, I found it to be super salty and prefer this version with baked goat cheese. It occurred to me this would make a really easy one-dish meal if you bake the fish along with the tomatoes. I love to use mini heirloom tomatoes, but there are a few options if you find yourself sensitive to tomatoes. First, try using tomatoes that aren't overly ripe. You can also remove the inner pulp to help lower glutamate levels, but since this is a challenge with smaller tomatoes, you can use beefsteak tomatoes and cut them into 1-inch chunks. If tomatoes aren't tolerated at all, this recipe also works with chopped roasted vegetables, especially assorted summer squash and broccoli. If you're not using tomatoes, I recommend balancing the missing acidity with a squeeze of fresh lemon juice to taste.

½ cup extra-virgin olive oil

One 4-ounce log soft goat cheese (chevre) or Boursin

1 pound mini heirloom tomatoes, or 1 pound (2 to 3 large) beefsteak tomatoes, seeds and pulp removed (see note above)

4 ounces asparagus, trimmed and cut into 2-inch pieces

2 whole garlic cloves

1 shallot, thinly sliced

Kosher salt and freshly ground black pepper

2 teaspoons chopped fresh oregano leaves

10 fresh basil leaves

1 pound halibut or other firm, flaky white fish, cut into 3 to 4 fillets, skin removed

8 ounces short pasta, such as rigatoni, farfalle, or penne, whole wheat or chickpea recommended

Preheat the oven to 400°F. Fill a large pot with salted water and set over high heat.

In a 3-quart baking dish, add olive oil and place goat cheese to one side. Add the tomatoes, asparagus, garlic, and shallot and toss with the olive oil. Sprinkle with a pinch of kosher salt and a few grinds of pepper. Add the oregano and 4 to 5 basil leaves. Put in the oven and bake until the goat cheese has softened all the way through, about 10 minutes. Nestle the halibut fillets in the pan, pushing the vegetables aside as needed. Return to the oven and bake until the halibut is just opaque at the center and flakes easily when tested with a knife, 14 to 17 minutes. Use a fork to smash the softened garlic cloves and mix them in with the rest of the vegetables.

Meanwhile, cook the pasta in the boiling water according to package directions until it is "al dente" (cooked through, but still firm to the bite in the center). Drain in a colander.

Carefully transfer the halibut fillets to a plate (a fish spatula can help). Add the pasta to the dish and, using a large spoon, mix together the vegetables, cheese, and pasta until incorporated. Place the halibut fillets on top of the mixture and sprinkle with remaining basil leaves, roughly torn.

To serve, spoon the pasta and halibut fillets into individual bowls.

Pan-Seared Salmon
with Warm Lentil Salad

MAKES 4 SERVINGS

A hearty meal, this simply seared salmon pairs perfectly with earthy
French lentils in a mustardy vegetable and thyme sauce. The lentil salad can be
prepped ahead and either served warm or at room temperature.

1½ cups French green lentils
(du Puy)

⅓ cup extra-virgin olive oil

1 cup chopped carrots

4 green onions, chopped

3 garlic cloves, minced

1 tablespoon distilled white
vinegar or lemon juice

1 tablespoon sulfite-free
Dijon mustard

¼ to ½ teaspoon dried thyme
leaves

Kosher salt and freshly ground
black pepper

1¾ pounds salmon fillets

2 teaspoons olive oil

Fresh parsley leaves for garnish

Fill a saucepan three-fourths full of water and bring to a boil over high
heat. Add the lentils, reduce the heat to medium, and simmer until
tender, 20 to 25 minutes. Drain and rinse the lentils and set aside.

In a large sauté pan over medium heat, warm the olive oil. Add the
carrots and sauté until softened, about 4 minutes. Add green onions
and garlic and sauté, stirring often so it doesn't burn, until everything
has softened, another 2 minutes. Pour the mixture into a bowl and add
the vinegar or lemon juice, mustard, and thyme leaves. Add the lentils
and toss to mix well. Taste and adjust the seasonings and keep warm.

Pat dry the salmon fillets and sprinkle lightly with kosher salt and
pepper. Wipe clean the sauté pan, then place over medium heat
with 2 teaspoons olive oil. Add the salmon to the pan flesh side down
and cook until it's lightly browned and releases from the pan easily,
4 to 5 minutes. Resist the urge to move the salmon while it cooks, as
this is how you get the nice golden-brown sear. Flip the salmon and
cook it skin side down until medium doneness, 4 to 5 minutes, or
until cooked through to your liking.

To serve, divide the warm lentil salad among serving plates and top
each with a salmon fillet. Top with fresh parsley leaves and serve
right away.

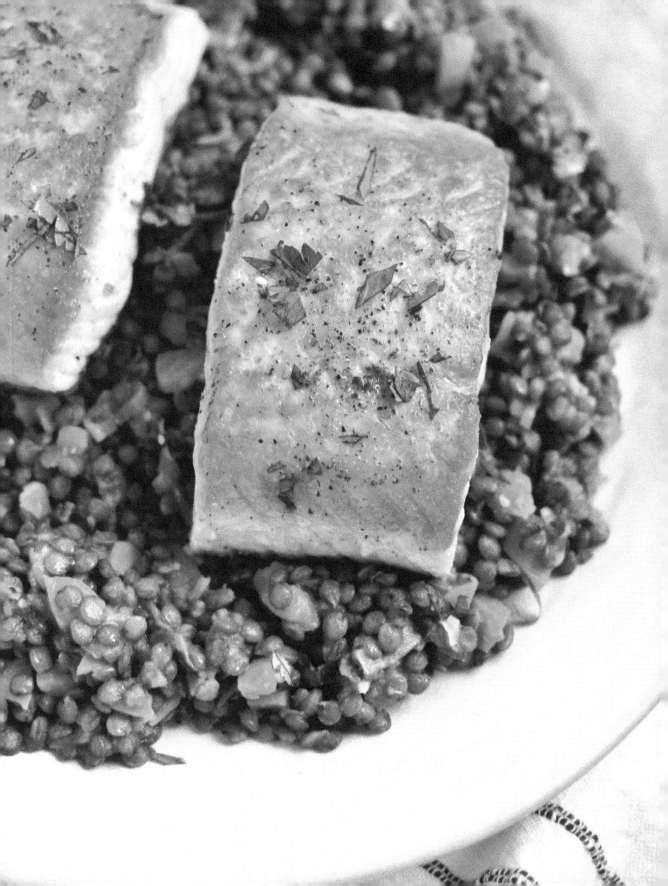

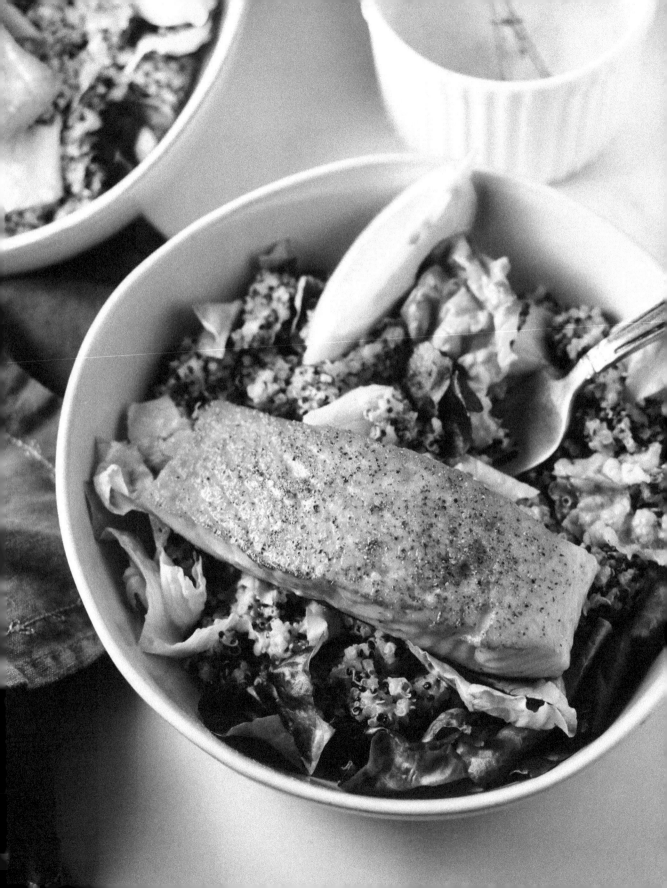

Salmon Salad Quinoa Bowl

MAKES 4 SERVINGS

While quinoa is a grain native to the Americas, it fits right in with a Mediterranean diet. Healthy and delicious, this bowl has my migraine-friendly dressing, which took quite a bit of time to develop to get the flavors just right. It can also be adjusted to be lower sodium. You can also use this dressing as a migraine-friendly substitution for Caesar dressing. For this recipe, I like to air-fry the salmon because it's a quick process for a weeknight meal. If you don't have an air fryer, see the Pan-Seared Salmon recipe on page 163 for instructions on how to cook salmon on the stove top.

---

1 cup water

1 cup vegetable broth

1 cup quinoa, rinsed

Olive oil spray

½ teaspoon salt

Four 4- to 6-ounce salmon fillets

TANGY GARLIC DRESSING

2 tablespoons mayonnaise

4 to 5 whole kalamata olives, pits removed and minced

1 large garlic clove, minced

1 tablespoon distilled white vinegar or ½ lemon, juiced

⅓ cup extra-virgin olive oil

Freshly ground black pepper

4 cups romaine lettuce, torn or cut into bite-sized pieces

In a saucepan, combine the water and broth and bring to a boil. Add the quinoa, cover, and reduce the heat to low. Simmer until the liquid is absorbed and the quinoa is light and fluffy, about 15 minutes. Turn off the heat but keep covered so it stays warm.

Following the manufacturer's instructions, heat the air fryer to 400°F. Spray the bottom of the air fryer with olive oil.

Season the salmon fillets with salt and pepper and place them skin side down in the air fryer basket. Cook until medium pink on the inside and golden brown on the top, 9 to 10 minutes, or until cooked to your liking.

While the salmon is cooking, make the dressing. In a bowl, whisk together the mayonnaise, olives, garlic, vinegar or lemon, olive oil, and a generous amount of pepper until smooth. Taste and adjust the seasonings.

Remove the salmon from the air-fryer. In a bowl, combine the quinoa, lettuce, and dressing and toss well. Divide the salad among serving bowls and top each with a salmon fillet.

TIP: For a low-sodium dressing, omit the olives. It won't have that same briny flavor but will still be delicious!

Herbed Shrimp-Stuffed Salmon

MAKES 4 SERVINGS

This is officially my favorite recipe when hosting friends and family. Any time I make this it gets a round of applause… and I almost feel guilty because it is so easy! It looks like you've spent all day in the kitchen, but it's ready in under 25 minutes. It's the ultimate sheet pan dinner, yet so impressive. I like to use frozen Argentinean shrimp (found at Trader Joe's or Costco) or langoustine tails, which are similar to lobster without the high price tag! However, you could easily use cooked lobster or crab as a substitute.

2 tablespoons extra-virgin olive oil

4 garlic cloves, minced

2 cups chopped raw peeled and deveined shrimp

4 ounces plain cream cheese

1 tablespoon soft goat cheese (chevre)

1 cup roughly torn spinach leaves

1 tablespoon chopped fresh basil

1 tablespoon chopped fresh parsley

Kosher salt and freshly ground black pepper

Four 6-ounce salmon fillets

Preheat the oven to 400°F. Line a large, rimmed baking sheet with parchment paper.

In a skillet, warm 1 tablespoon of the olive oil over medium heat. Add the garlic and cook, stirring often, until soft and fragrant but not brown, about 1 minute. Add the chopped shrimp and cook, stirring often, until just opaque, 2 to 3 minutes. Turn off the heat and mix in the cream cheese, goat cheese, spinach, basil, and parsley until incorporated. Taste and adjust any seasonings.

Pat the salmon dry with a paper towel. Arrange the salmon fillets skin side down on the prepared baking sheet and drizzle with the remaining 1 tablespoon of oil. Make a ½-inch slit deep into the center of each fillet and pull the slit open to create space to stuff the shrimp mixture. Season the fillets with salt and pepper. Spoon the shrimp mixture into each of the slits, dividing evenly, allowing the filling to spill out a bit on top of the fillets. Bake until the flesh is cooked medium, and the filling is hot, 15 to 18 minutes or until cooked to your liking.

Divide the stuffed fillets among serving plates and serve warm.

NOTE: For a dairy-free dish, omit the cheeses and add ¼ cup dried breadcrumbs to the stuffing mixture.

TIP: For an easy side dish, toss 1 pound of trimmed asparagus spears with 2 teaspoons olive oil and arrange on a baking sheet. Roast the asparagus alongside the fish for the same amount of time, then season to your preference.

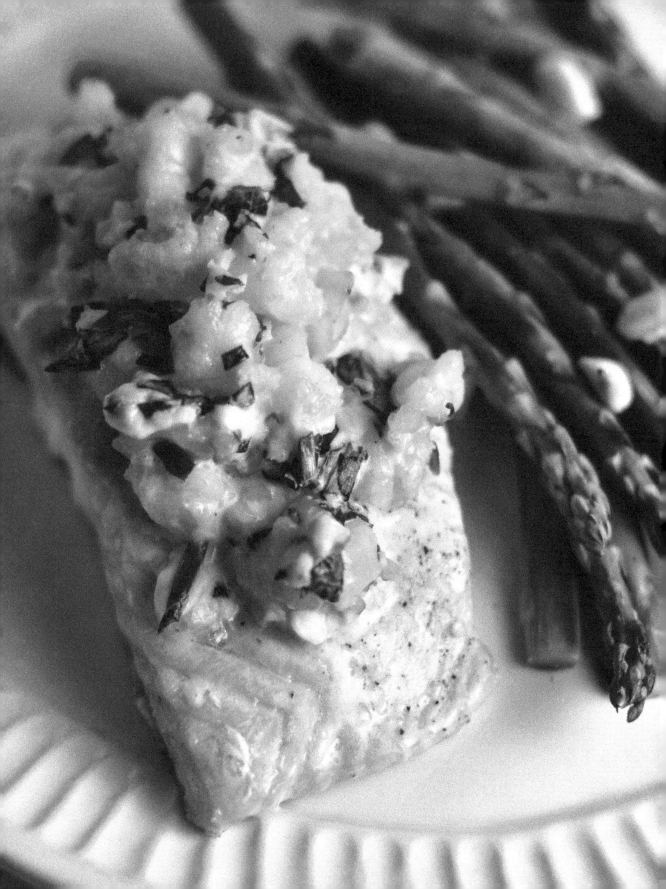

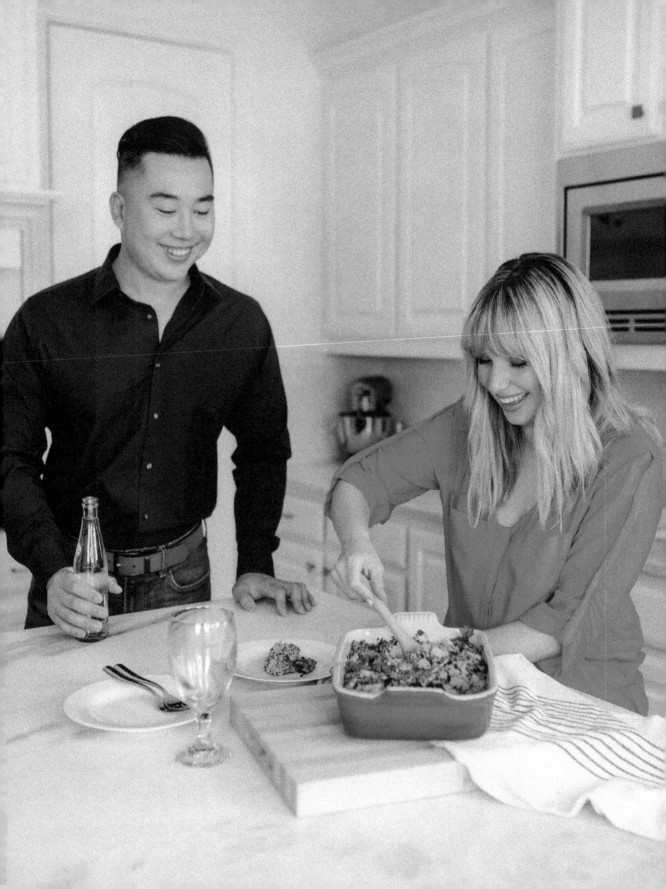

POULTRY

THE BENEFITS OF POULTRY

Records from 600 BC show the ancient Babylonians enjoying chicken meat. Today, chicken is undoubtedly the most widely farmed source of animal protein. It is cheap, versatile, and used in almost every culture. Chicken meat is low in saturated fat (after trimming away the skin and all visible fat) and is a healthy source of protein.

Duck has a unique and rich flavor, which pairs well with naturally sweet fruits and vegetables. Duck has a lot of fat beneath the skin to help ducks float and stay warm, but if the skin and visible fat are trimmed, the meat is very lean. Duck fat has a lower saturated fat percentage compared to beef or pork, but it has more saturated fat compared to extra-virgin olive oil.

SHOPPING FOR POULTRY

When buying poultry, it's important to read the labels. You might be asking, why would they add anything to raw meat? You'd be surprised that it happens all the time. One of the most important things I learned from my butcher about choosing chicken was to always look for "Air Chilled." "Air-chilled is more important to how chicken cooks and tastes than organic is," he told me. Whether roasting, grilling, or pan-searing, I find this to be true.

Conventional chicken or turkey can be dunked into or injected with a water solution during chilling. This causes the meat to absorb some of the solution, which can alter the flavor and texture. These same solutions have the potential to trigger a migraine attack. Air-chilled poultry, on the other hand, is passed through chambers of cold air to properly cool the poultry to the right temperature. It doesn't take on excess moisture and is perfect for roasting and grilling. Air-chilled poultry is also great for migraine patients wary of the solutions that are added to make birds plumper—these same solutions can trigger a migraine attack.

Rosemary extract is another ingredient that's often included with turkey to slow oxidation, and not a common trigger ingredient, but be mindful to check for of any broths or "natural flavorings," especially if you're sensitive to MSG.

If you choose to buy organic poultry, by all means, do so. But it's not necessary to eat organic simply to be "migraine friendly." What's most important is making sure your chicken only contains chicken.

Coastal Chicken Salad

MAKES 4 SERVINGS

I am a chicken salad aficionado. I love a good chicken salad and I'm a huge fan of savory and sweet combinations. This might remind you of the classic Waldorf salad, which uses so many fresh fruits and vegetables that fit into the Mediterranean diet. It's perfect to enjoy for a warm day on the coast... or in your own backyard! Serve on toasted whole-grain bread for a sandwich, with crackers as a salad, or with endive leaves to scoop it up. To make this easy, buy a "naked" rotisserie chicken (a chicken seasoned only with salt, pepper, and olive oil) from a local market. They can be found at Fresh Market, Sprouts, and Whole Foods, just to name a few. I prefer honeycrisp apples for their sweetness, but any favorite apple will work here.

3 cups diced cooked chicken breast (about 1 pound)

1 cup red grapes, quartered

1 cup chopped honeycrisp apples

⅓ cup celery, chopped

⅓ cup mayonnaise

1 teaspoon poppy seeds

½ teaspoon freshly ground black pepper

¼ cup toasted, unsalted pumpkin seeds (pepitas)

In a large bowl, combine the chicken, grapes, apples, celery, mayonnaise, poppy seeds, and pepper and mix gently but thoroughly. Chill for at least 20 minutes to let the flavors meld. This can be stored, tightly covered in the refrigerator, for 3 to 4 days.

Just before serving, mix in the pumpkin seeds.

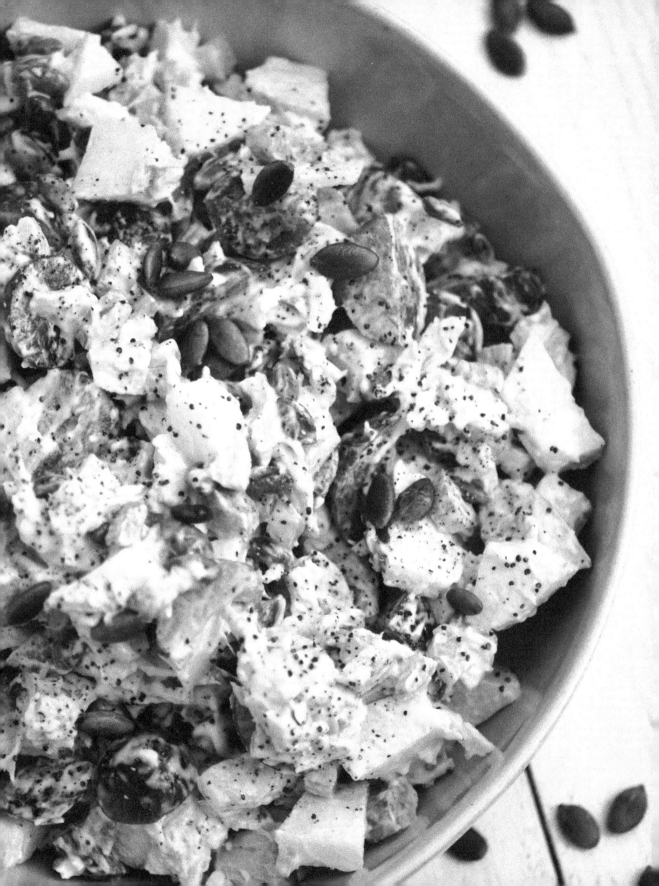

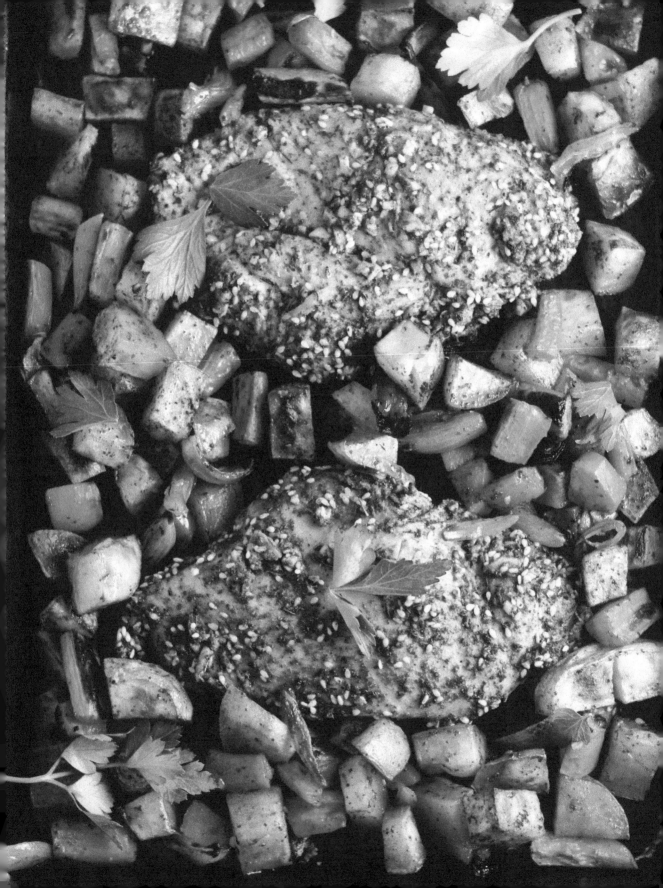

Za'atar Roast Chicken
with Sumac Potatoes & Carrots

SERVES 4

Za'atar, a Middle Eastern spice mixture typically containing cumin, oregano, thyme, coriander, and sesame seeds, is one of my favorite spice blends. It is widely available at many grocery stores these days—even Target and Trader Joe's. If you still cannot find it, there are so many easy recipes online and I promise it will be used again! Za'atar pairs beautifully with poultry, roasted vegetables, and hummus. This recipe was inspired by one on my website that uses a whole chicken, but I simplified it here for a weeknight dinner. These roasted chicken breasts are juicy, and pair well with the carrots and potatoes for a flavorful, complete dinner. I recommend investing in a meat thermometer, which will help to avoid overcooking and drying out the chicken breasts.

SUMAC POTATOES & CARROTS

3 to 4 Yukon gold potatoes, cut into chunks

3 large carrots, peeled and cut into large chunks

2 to 3 shallots, peeled and cut into wedges

1 tablespoon olive oil

1 teaspoon sumac

Kosher salt and freshly ground black pepper

ZA'ATAR CHICKEN

2 pounds boneless, skinless chicken breasts

2 teaspoons olive oil

2 garlic cloves, minced

2½ tablespoons za'atar

Kosher salt and freshly ground black pepper

Fresh parsley leaves for garnish

To make the Sumac Potatoes and Carrots, preheat the oven to 400°F. In a large, rimmed baking sheet toss the potato wedges, carrots, and shallots with the olive oil, sumac, and salt and pepper to taste (I typically start with ½ teaspoon). Spread everything out in a single layer. Roast for 15 minutes.

To make the Za'atar Chicken, use a mallet (or your hand) to pound the chicken breasts to about ½ inch thickness. Place them in a bowl with the olive oil, garlic, za'atar, and a pinch of salt and pepper. Stir until well coated.

Remove the baking sheet from the oven. Toss the vegetables and make two spaces for the chicken breasts. Place the chicken breasts on the sheet pan and return to the oven. Roast until the vegetables are tender and golden and the center of the chicken registers 165°F when tested on a meat thermometer, 20 to 25 minutes.

Remove from oven, taste and adjust any seasonings, and serve warm garnished with parsley leaves.

Fattoush Salad
with Chicken & Grilled Halloumi

MAKES 4 SERVINGS

One of my favorite Mediterranean recipes is the fattoush salad—a mix of greens, cucumber, sumac, and pita bread. Paired with easy grilled chicken (which I make almost weekly for meal prep) and salty halloumi cheese, it's a healthy and protein-rich meal. This is the kind of recipe you can switch up. For a low sodium dish, switch to a fresh cheese like goat cheese. Please don't skip the sumac! It's used in lots of recipes in this cookbook and is a tough flavor to replace. The chicken, vegetables, and halloumi can all be made ahead and assembled before serving. I recommend waiting to grill the pita at the last minute, so it remains warm with a bit of crunch.

MARINATED CHICKEN

2 chicken breasts

¼ cup mustard (I used Dijon)

2 garlic cloves, minced

1 tablespoon extra-virgin olive oil

½ teaspoon kosher salt

¼ teaspoon black pepper

SUMAC VINAIGRETTE

⅓ cup extra-virgin olive oil

3 tablespoons lemon juice or distilled white vinegar

1 teaspoon sumac

¼ teaspoon paprika

1 garlic clove, minced

½ teaspoon honey

CONTINUED ON PAGE 179

To marinate the chicken, in a shallow dish, combine the chicken, mustard, garlic, olive oil, salt, and pepper, and stir to fully coat the chicken. Cover and refrigerate for at least 1 hour, up to 24 hours.

To make the sumac vinaigrette, in a bowl, combine the olive oil, lemon juice, sumac, paprika, garlic, and honey. Whisk until smooth and the olive oil is fully incorporated (no separation). Cover and store in the refrigerator until ready to serve.

When the chicken has marinated, prepare the fattoush salad. Preheat a gas grill or stovetop grill pan to medium-high heat. Lay the eggplant rounds on a baking sheet and lightly season with salt. Allow them to sit for 5 to 10 minutes to draw out moisture, then blot both sides with a paper towel. Brush the eggplant, halloumi, and pita with olive oil on both sides.

CONTINUED ON PAGE 179

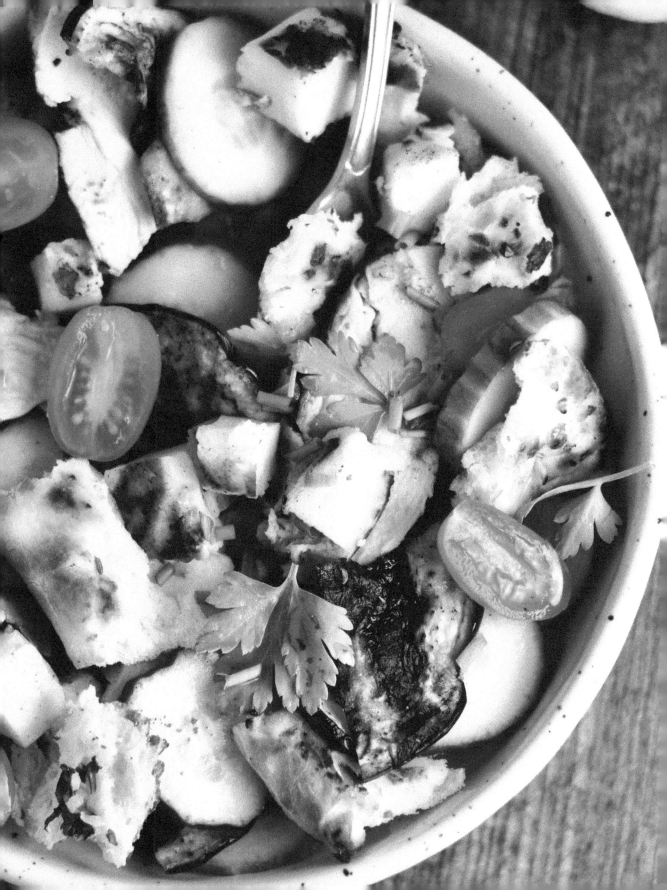

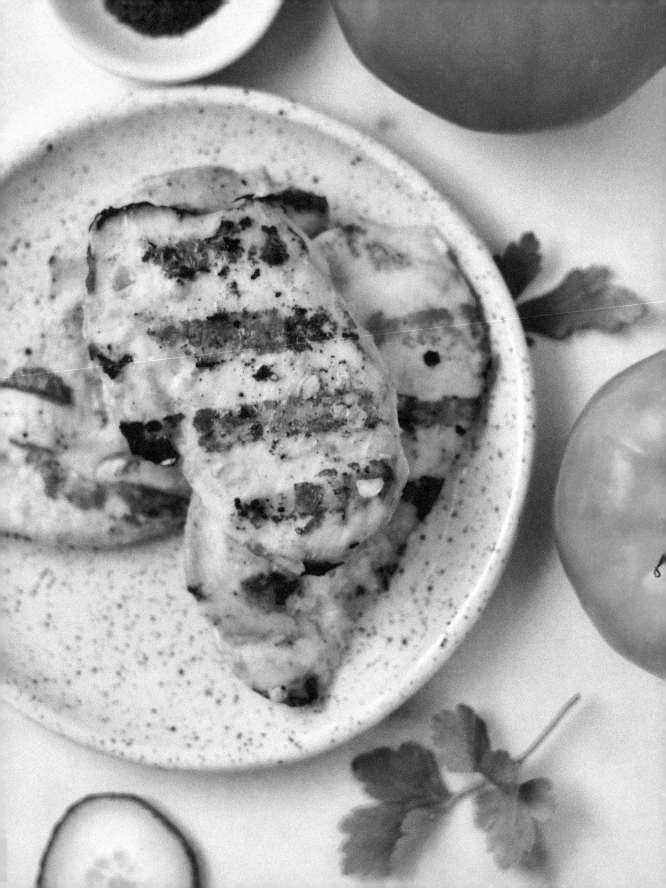

Fattoush Salad with Chicken & Grilled Halloumi (continued)

FATTOUSH SALAD

1 small eggplant, sliced into ¼-inch rounds

Kosher salt and freshly ground black pepper to taste

8 ounces halloumi cheese, sliced in half

2 pita breads

2 tablespoons extra-virgin olive oil (for brushing eggplant, pita, and halloumi)

1 romaine lettuce heart, roughly chopped

8 ounces tomatoes, finely chopped (I recommend cherry or beefsteak tomatoes with seeds and pulp removed, depending on tolerance)

1 cup chopped English (seedless) cucumber

¼ cup fresh parsley leaves

1 tablespoon fresh mint leaves (optional)

When the grill is hot, add the chicken, eggplant, pita, and halloumi to the grates, leaving a sheet pan next to it to remove food as it is ready. Close the grill lid (if not using a grill pan). Grill the chicken breasts until grill marks form and it reaches an internal temperature of 165°F, about 8 minutes per side. Grill the eggplant rounds until softened and grill marks have formed, about 6 minutes per side. Grill the halloumi until grill marks have formed, 2 to 3 minutes per side. Grill the pita, flipping once, until warmed through with some grill marks, 3 to 4 minutes total. Remove everything from the grill as it is ready and set it aside on the baking sheet.

When everything has been grilled, cut the chicken into slices. Cut the halloumi into cubes. Tear the pita into bite-size pieces.

In a large bowl, combine the chicken, eggplant, pita, halloumi, romaine lettuce, tomatoes, cucumber, parsley, and mint leaves, if using. Toss everything with a few tablespoons of sumac vinaigrette, tasting and adjusting the dressing to your preference. Sprinkle with salt and fresh black pepper to finish. Serve right away.

NOTE: For a dairy-free salad, leave out the halloumi. For a plant-based dish, omit the chicken and bread and enjoy as a simple salad.

Chicken & Artichoke Casserole

MAKES 4 SERVINGS

This is a recipe my family asks for on repeat. A one-dish casserole, it's filled with lots of great vegetables and a very light Boursin sauce. Although this could be made with brown rice, I often like to reach for protein-rich quinoa. This is a wonderful recipe to reheat the next day or keep on hand for lunch. I think it would be a great one to make for a friend or family in need!

---

1 cup quinoa, rinsed

3 cups vegetable or chicken broth

Olive oil

1 pound boneless, skinless chicken breasts, cut into bite-size pieces

Kosher salt and freshly ground black pepper

3 garlic cloves, minced

⅓ cup chopped shallot

One 14-ounce can artichokes, rinsed, drained, and chopped

2 teaspoons cornstarch or all-purpose flour

½ cup milk

1 cup fresh spinach leaves

½ package Boursin Garlic and Fine Herbs cheese

In a covered pot, combine the quinoa with 2 cups of the broth and bring to a boil over high heat. Reduce the heat to low and simmer until all the liquid is absorbed and the grains are fluffy, 15 to 20 minutes.

Preheat the oven to 375°F and oil a 9-by-13-inch baking dish.

Season the chicken with salt and pepper. In a large skillet over medium heat, warm 2 teaspoons olive oil. Add the chicken pieces and cook until golden brown on all sides, about 5 minutes total. Transfer the chicken to a plate and set aside.

In the same pan over medium heat, warm another 2 teaspoons olive oil. Add the garlic and shallots and cook, stirring often with a wooden spoon so garlic does not burn, until softened and fragrant, about 2 minutes. Add the artichokes and cornstarch or flour. Slowly stir in the remaining 1 cup broth and the milk, whisking until the mixture is smooth and the cornstarch or flour is fully combined. Simmer, stirring often with a wooden spoon, until the sauce has thickened, about 5 minutes. Reduce the heat to low and stir in the spinach leaves and cheese, mixing until smooth. Add the chicken and quinoa and stir well.

Pour the chicken mixture into the prepared baking dish and bake until warm throughout and lightly browned on top, about 20 minutes.

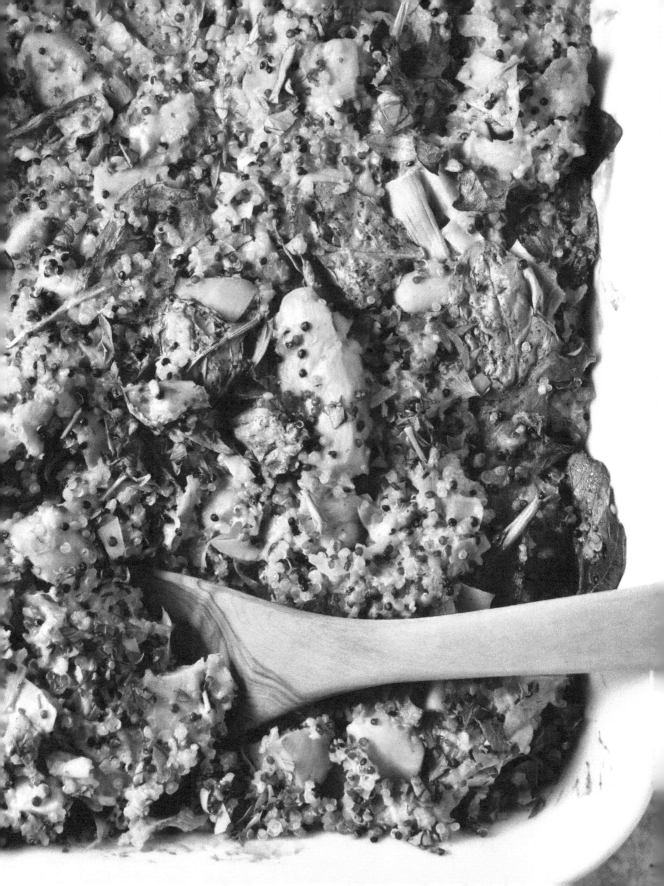

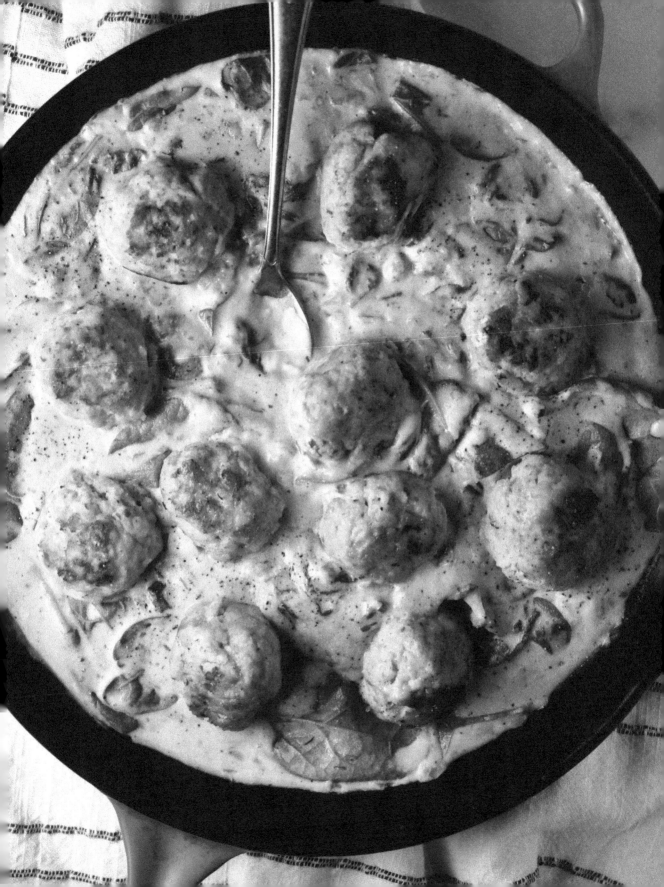

Chicken Meatballs with Creamy Spinach Sauce

MAKES 10 MEATBALLS

Serve these savory meatballs coated in a spinach-flecked cheese sauce with a light salad and potatoes, rice, or quinoa to soak up the sauce. For best results, I recommend using whole milk because it stands up well to heat without curdling. You can use a lower fat version; just be careful so that it doesn't boil, keeping the heat low at all times and stirring the sauce frequently. I also recommend letting the milk come to room temperature before using.

1 pound ground chicken or turkey

2 cloves garlic, minced

¼ cup panko

1 teaspoon dried Mediterranean oregano

1 shallot, chopped (about ⅓ cup)

Kosher salt and freshly ground black pepper

1 tablespoon extra-virgin olive oil

1 tablespoon all-purpose flour

1 cup vegetable or chicken broth

1 cup milk

2 teaspoons Dijon mustard

2 ounces cream cheese

2 cups spinach leaves

In a small bowl, combine the ground chicken, garlic, panko, oregano, shallot, ½ teaspoon salt, and about ¼ teaspoon black pepper and mix until thoroughly combined. Using your hands, form the mixture into 10 meatballs and place on a plate.

In a large skillet over medium heat, warm the olive oil. Add the meatballs and cook until golden brown on all sides and cooked through, turning as needed, 9 to 10 minutes total. For extra assurance, insert an instant-read thermometer into the center of a meatball; it should register 165°F. Put the meatballs on a clean plate and set aside.

Add the flour to the same pan over low heat, and use a wooden spoon to stir it into the drippings. Whisk in the broth until well blended and smooth. Stir in the milk. Bring the mixture to a low simmer over medium-high heat, and cook until the sauce has thickened enough to coat the spoon, 5 to 7 minutes. Reduce the heat to low and stir in the mustard and cream cheese. Taste and adjust any seasonings.

Add the spinach to the pan and stir over low heat until the leaves are wilted, 1 to 2 minutes. Add the meatballs to the sauce and cook, stirring occasionally, until everything is heated through, 1 to 2 minutes.

Divide the meatballs and sauce among shallow bowls and serve warm.

NOTE: For a dairy-free dish, use unsweetened oat milk and omit the cheese. For a gluten-free dish, use gluten-free panko and gluten-free all-purpose flour.

Rosemary Chicken & Rice Casserole

MAKES 4 SERVINGS

One of my favorite full-dinner meals, this dish is filling and delicious, featuring simple ingredients and lots of vegetables. It reheats well and would make a great dish for meal prepping. I used Lundberg Wild Rice Blend for the rice. You could use all brown rice, but the texture and taste of the blend is much more elevated. I use chicken thighs here for extra flavor, but chicken breast can be substituted with the same cooking time. Just wait to add them back into the mixture until the sauce has cooked through or they may dry out.

---

1 cup wild rice blend

Water or broth as needed

2 tablespoons extra virgin olive oil

1½ pounds boneless, skinless chicken thighs, cut into bite-sized pieces

Kosher salt and freshly ground black pepper

½ cup chopped carrots

½ cup chopped shallots

½ cup chopped apples (I used honeycrisp)

1½ cups vegetable or chicken broth

2 tablespoons sulfite-free Dijon mustard

1 tablespoon minced fresh rosemary leaves, plus leaves for garnish

½ teaspoon dried thyme leaves

2 tablespoons heavy cream (optional)

In a saucepan, cook the wild rice according to package directions. For the best flavor, I recommend using ½ broth and ½ water for the liquid.

Meanwhile in a large, heavy skillet over medium heat, heat 1 tablespoon of olive oil. Add the chicken pieces, season lightly with salt and pepper, and cook until browned on all sides and just cooked through, 6 to 7 minutes. Increase the heat as needed to get the chicken nicely browned. Transfer the chicken to a plate.

To the same pan over medium heat, add the remaining olive oil. Add the carrots, shallots, apples, and a pinch of salt and pepper and sauté until softened, 5 to 6 minutes. Pour in the 1½ cups broth, scraping any browned bits from the bottom of the pan, and bring to a boil. Reduce the heat to low and add the cooked chicken, mustard, rosemary, and thyme, and simmer until the liquid is reduced, about 5 minutes. If using, add the heavy cream and simmer for another 5 minutes (10 minutes total). The sauce will be just slightly thickened. Taste and adjust the seasonings.

In a large serving bowl, layer the cooked rice, chicken, and sauce. Garnish with rosemary and serve right away.

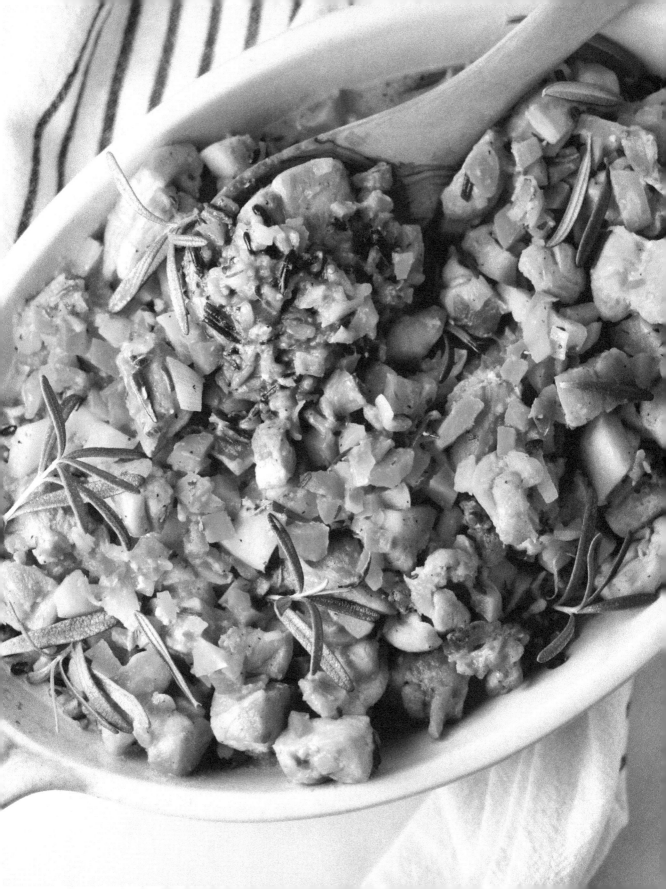

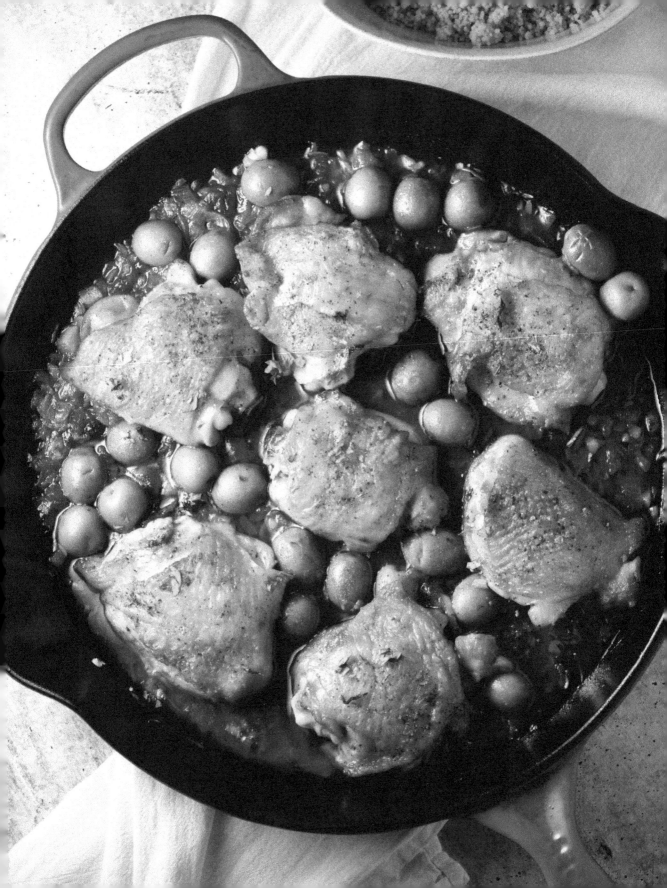

Roasted Olive Chicken with Couscous

MAKES 4 SERVINGS

This Moroccan-inspired dish is delicious and flavorful with the sweetness from the apricots mixed with briny olives and savory, crispy-skinned chicken thighs. It's amazing served with quick-cooking couscous. Be sure to choose apricots without sulfites (they'll be an awful brown color, but that's a good thing!) and Castelvetrano olives with pits packed in water. Navigating the olive pits while eating is a mild inconvenience, but olives with pits are not processed as much as pitted. I've found that this makes them more tolerable for some people who are sensitive to olives.

CHICKEN

2 pounds bone-in, skin-on chicken thighs (4 or 5 large pieces)

Kosher salt and freshly ground black pepper

1 tablespoon extra-virgin olive oil

2 large shallots, chopped

4 cloves garlic, minced

½ teaspoon ground cumin

½ teaspoon paprika

¼ teaspoon ground turmeric

¼ teaspoon ground ginger

⅓ cup sulfite-free dried apricots, chopped

1 cup vegetable or chicken broth

½ cup Castelvetrano olives

COUSCOUS

1 cup vegetable or chicken broth

1 tablespoon olive oil

1 cup durum wheat couscous

Kosher salt and freshly ground black pepper

Preheat the oven to 400°F.

Pat dry the chicken thighs and season lightly with salt and pepper. In an oven-safe skillet or cast-iron pan over medium high heat, warm the 1 tablespoon olive oil. Add the chicken thighs skin down and sear 5 minutes. Don't mess with them! After 5 minutes, check to see if it's golden brown, adjusting the heat as necessary. If they're not ready to be turned, let sear for another minute or two. Flip the chicken and cook on the other side in the same manner. The chicken does not need to be cooked through at this point. Transfer the browned chicken to a plate.

Reduce the heat to medium-low. To the same pan, add the shallots, garlic, cumin, paprika, turmeric, and ginger and cook, stirring often, until fragrant and warmed through, about 1 minute. Add the apricots and broth and bring to a simmer. Return the chicken to the pan and scatter the olives around. Place the pan in the oven and bake until the chicken is cooked through and reads 165°F on a meat thermometer, about 10 minutes.

Meanwhile, to make the couscous, in a saucepan, bring the 1 cup of broth to a boil with the 1 tablespoon olive oil. Stir in the couscous, cover, and turn off heat. Let the couscous stand until the liquid is absorbed, about 10 minutes. Uncover the pan, fluff the grains with a fork, and season to taste with salt and pepper.

To serve, divide the couscous among serving plates and top with the chicken and sauce.

Seared Duck with Cherry Sauce

MAKES 4 SERVINGS

Duck doesn't just have to be for special occasions at fancy restaurants—it's really easy to cook at home! This sweet and savory, Italian-style cherry sauce cuts the richness of the duck meat. Remember: Don't throw away the duck fat when you're done cooking! Store it in an airtight container in the freezer for up to one year. If you're sensitive to cured meat like bacon, duck fat is a fantastic substitute for that rich flavor in dishes that call for it. This dish pairs well with wild or brown rice or mashed cauliflower.

---

24 frozen pitted cherries (about 1 heaping cup)

½ cup vegetable broth

¼ cup unsweetened apple juice

2 teaspoons distilled white vinegar

4 boneless duck breasts, about 5 ounces each

1 shallot, chopped

2 tablespoons honey

Kosher salt and freshly ground black pepper

Put the frozen cherries, broth, apple juice, and vinegar in a bowl and let the cherries soak (they will thaw a bit during this time).

Using a sharp knife, score the skin of the duck breasts in a crosshatch pattern, being careful to not cut through to the meat. The deeper you cut, the more fat that will render off the breast while cooking. Season the duck all over with salt and pepper.

Place the duck breasts skin-side down in a large skillet. Turn on the heat to medium-low and allow it to start to sizzle, which should begin after 2 to 3 minutes. If you don't hear that sound, increase the heat to medium. Cook the duck breasts undisturbed until the skin is golden brown and the internal temperature registers 125°F when tested with a meat thermometer, 13 to 15 minutes.

Flip the duck breasts and cook until the internal temperature reaches 130° to 140°F for medium-rare to medium, 4 to 5 minutes. Transfer the duck to a plate. Drain the excess fat in the pan into an empty can or a container that will hold hot oil, leaving about 1 tablespoon behind.

Place the pan with the duck fat over medium heat. Add the shallot and sauté until softened, 1 to 2 minutes. Add the cherry-broth mixture along with the honey and bring to a boil. Cook, stirring often, until the liquid is slightly reduced, 8 to 10 minutes. The sauce should thicken and become sticky enough to coat a spoon.

Remove the sauce from the heat. Taste to adjust the seasonings. When ready to serve, slice the duck against the grain into ½-inch pieces and divide among serving plates. Spoon the cherry sauce over the top and serve right away.

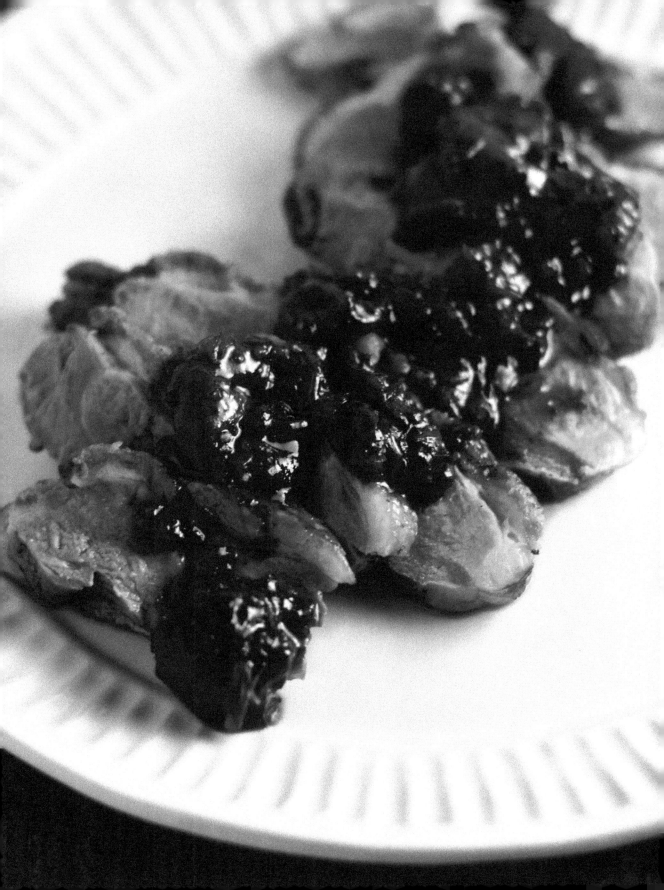

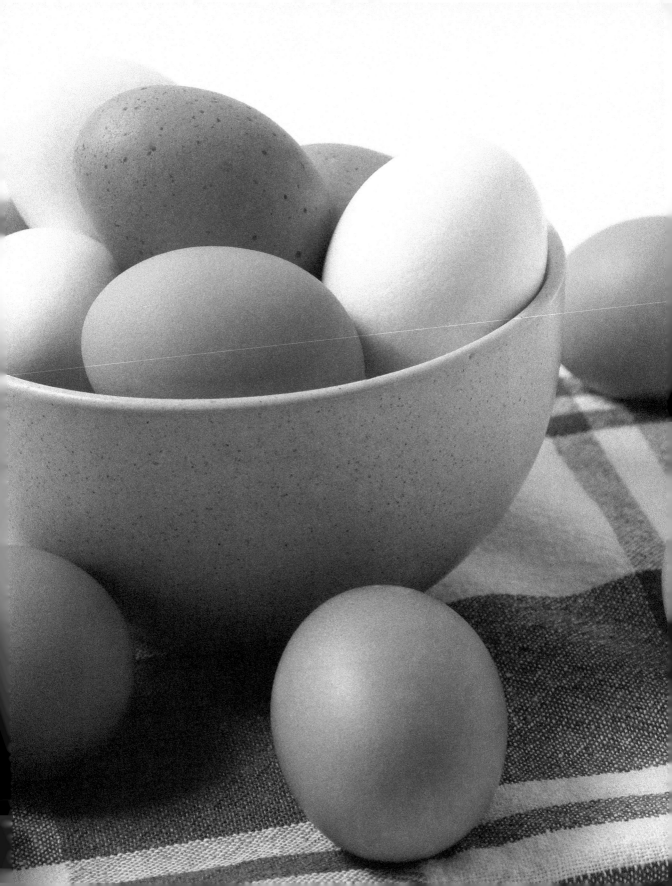

EGGS

THE BENEFITS OF EGGS

Eggs are an inexpensive, versatile, and convenient protein source that provides vitamins B2, B6, B12, D, and E. Omega-3 enriched eggs are from chickens that are fed flaxseed. Eggs are easy to prepare, and can be used to make healthy meals or snacks to ensure those with migraine maintain a consistent eating schedule, which can help prevent symptoms from appearing.

SHOPPING FOR EGGS

Eggs can be a tricky topic when it comes to migraine. They're so good for you, yet I hear enough complaints from Dizzy Cook readers about them being a trigger to have looked into why this could be. What I've found is that where you buy eggs and what type you buy can really make a difference for people who are egg sensitive.

One of the biggest issues seems to be that soy is often included in the hen's diets, and some people with migraine are sensitive to soy. Pasture-raised, organic eggs are always preferable, but folks who are sensitive to eggs may want to seek out soy-free eggs.

When looking for these at the grocery store, they're usually not the fancy, flashy boxes, but simply labeled "soy free." I've found them at Whole Foods and Central Market. If you source your eggs from a local farm or farmers' market, ask them what they put in the feed—you can often find it on the brand's website.

Finally, having chickens has become a trend here in Texas. A friend in my ballet class brings us extra eggs from her backyard hens—delicious! If you can find yourself a friend that raises chickens, that's even better.

Broccoli Artichoke Quiche Cups

MAKES 12 MINI QUICHES

Muffin-pan quiches are one of my favorite make-ahead recipes because they make a
great grab-and-go breakfast and freeze well. Somehow, I find them easier to make than
a whole quiche! You can use your favorite homemade pie dough recipe or save some time
by using a favorite store-bought pie dough. While I love this recipe without cheese,
I will occasionally add ¼ cup of mozzarella or soft goat cheese.

Olive oil or butter

5 large eggs

½ cup milk

⅔ cup finely chopped
broccoli florets

4 artichoke hearts, chopped
(about ⅓ cup)

½ teaspoon minced fresh
rosemary

½ teaspoon kosher salt

¼ teaspoon freshly ground
black pepper

Flour, for rolling

Prepared pie dough for a
9-inch pie crust (unbaked),
at room temperature

Preheat the oven to 375°F. Grease the cups of a 12-cup muffin pan
with olive oil or butter.

In a bowl, combine the eggs, milk, broccoli, artichoke hearts, rosemary,
salt, and pepper and whisk until light and fluffy.

Place the pie dough on a lightly floured work surface. Using a rolling
pin, roll out the dough into a round as thin as possible, ⅛- to ¼-inch
thick. Using a large cup or round cookie cutter, cut out 12 circles
about 3 inches in diameter. Place a dough round in the bottom of each
muffin cup—the dough doesn't need to go all the way up to the top.
Using the tines of a fork, poke several holes in the bottom and sides
of the crusts. Pour about ¼ cup of the egg mixture into each muffin
cup. Transfer the pan to the oven and bake until the quiches are lightly
browned on top, 23 to 27 minutes.

Remove the quiches from the oven and allow them to cool in the pan
about 5 minutes. Then, slide a knife along the edge of each muffin cup
and carefully lift out the quiches.

Serve warm or let cool and store in the refrigerator for up to 3 days or
in the freezer for up to 4 months.

NOTES: For dairy-free quiches, substitute oat milk for dairy milk. For
gluten-free quiches, use gluten-free pie dough. Or you can make these
without a crust by oiling the muffin cups thoroughly and reducing the
cooking time to 15 to 20 minutes.

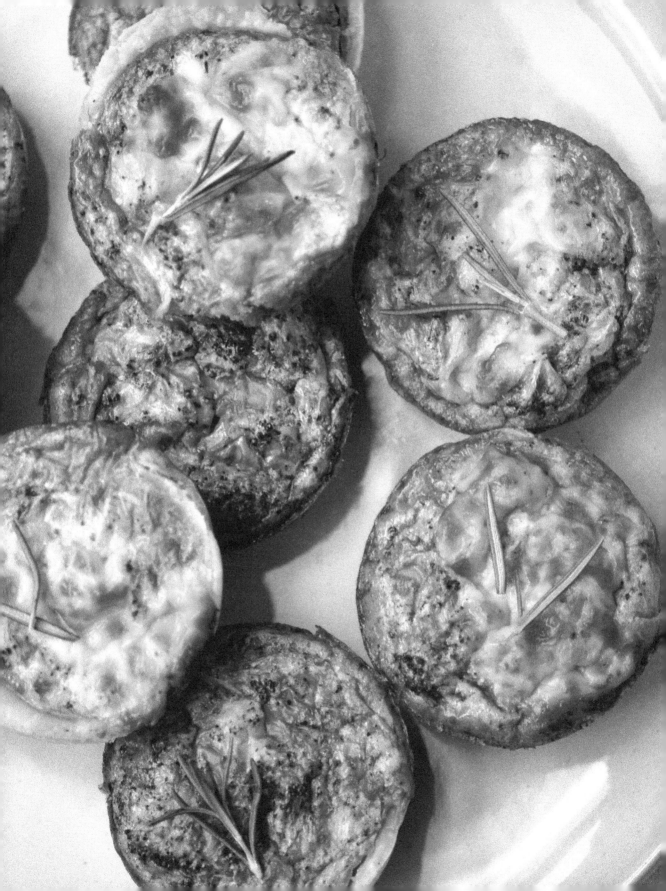

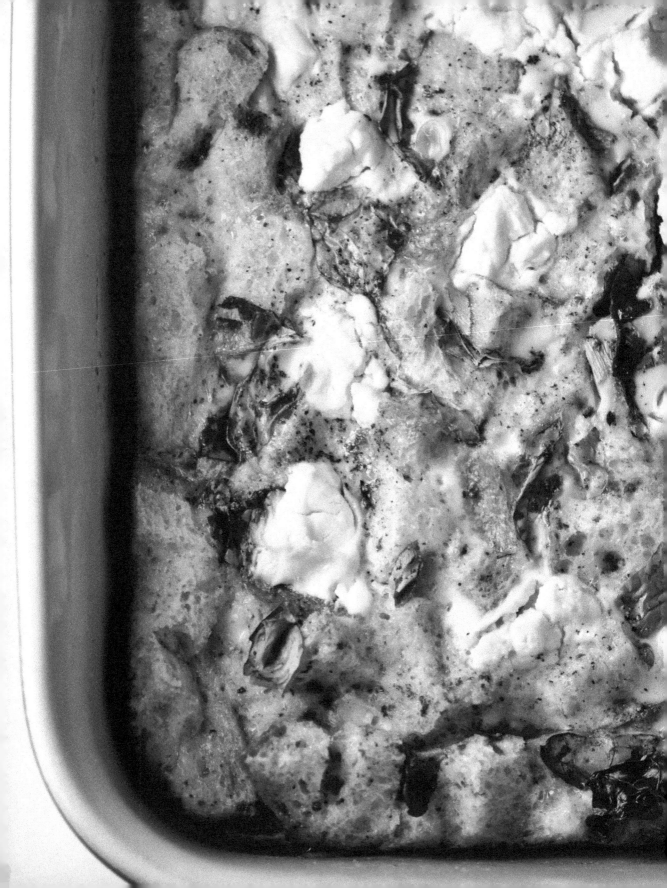

Super-Easy Egg Casserole

MAKES 6 TO 8 SERVINGS

This dish is inspired by a strata, which I've modified for a Mediterranean diet by decreasing the amount of bread used, and opting for whole-grain bread. I find this balance to be more egg focused with just enough bread to make it crunchy in spots. The spices add a lot of great flavor and pair well with the cheese and spinach. Use any kind of milk you prefer in this recipe.

Olive oil spray

5 slices multigrain or whole-wheat bread, cut into cubes

11 large eggs

2 green onions, chopped (about ½ cup)

¾ cup milk

3 ounces soft goat cheese or herbed cream cheese

½ teaspoon garlic powder

½ teaspoon paprika

¼ teaspoon dried marjoram

¼ teaspoon dried sage powder

1 cup torn spinach leaves

½ teaspoon kosher salt

¼ teaspoon freshly ground black pepper

Preheat oven to 350°F. Spray a 9-by-13-inch baking pan with olive oil.

Scatter the cubed bread on the bottom of the prepared baking pan. In a bowl, combine the eggs, green onions, milk, cheese, garlic powder, paprika, marjoram, sage, and spinach and whisk until smooth. Pour the mixture over the bread and sprinkle with the salt and pepper. Bake until the eggs are fully cooked, and the top is light golden, 15 to 20 minutes.

You can bake this up to 24 hours in advance or freeze after baking (up to three months) and reheat in the microwave or oven.

Tarragon Egg Salad

MAKES 2 TO 3 SERVINGS

Tarragon has a licorice or anise flavor that can be strong, but somehow it just works
in this recipe without being overpowering. It's important the tarragon is fresh and not dried.
My favorite way to serve is layered on toast with a little extra chopped tarragon
sprinkled on top. Unfortunately, Greek yogurt is a personal food trigger for me,
but it could be used as a mayonnaise substitute here for a tangier flavor!

6 large eggs

1 small shallot, chopped
(about 2 tablespoons)

1 tablespoon minced
fresh tarragon

2 teaspoons dried chives
or 1 tablespoon chopped
fresh chives

¼ cup mayonnaise

1 teaspoon distilled
white vinegar

Kosher salt and pepper

Bring a saucepan of water to a boil over high heat. Prepare a large bowl
of ice water.

Using a spoon, carefully add the eggs to the boiling water so they
don't crack. Boil the eggs for 11 to 12 minutes. Using a slotted spoon,
pull the eggs out of the boiling water and plunge them into ice water
to stop the cooking.

When the eggs have cooled, peel them, discarding the eggshells and
placing the eggs in a bowl. Using a fork, mash the eggs well. Add the
shallot, tarragon, chives, mayonnaise, and vinegar. Stir with the fork
until fully combined, then add kosher salt and pepper to taste.

Serve right away or make ahead and store in the refrigerator up
to three days.

TIP: If you can't find fresh tarragon, fresh basil is also delicious.

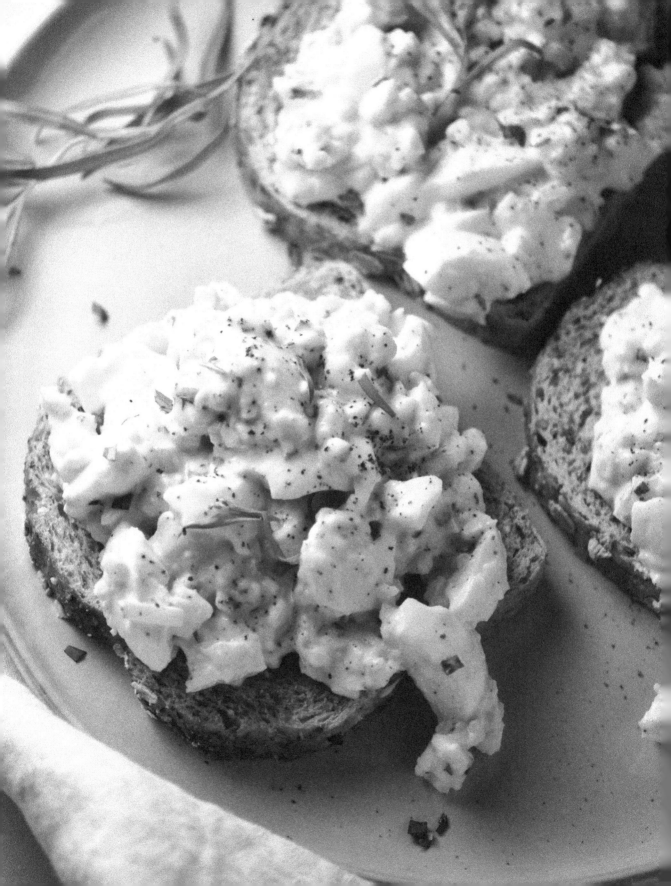

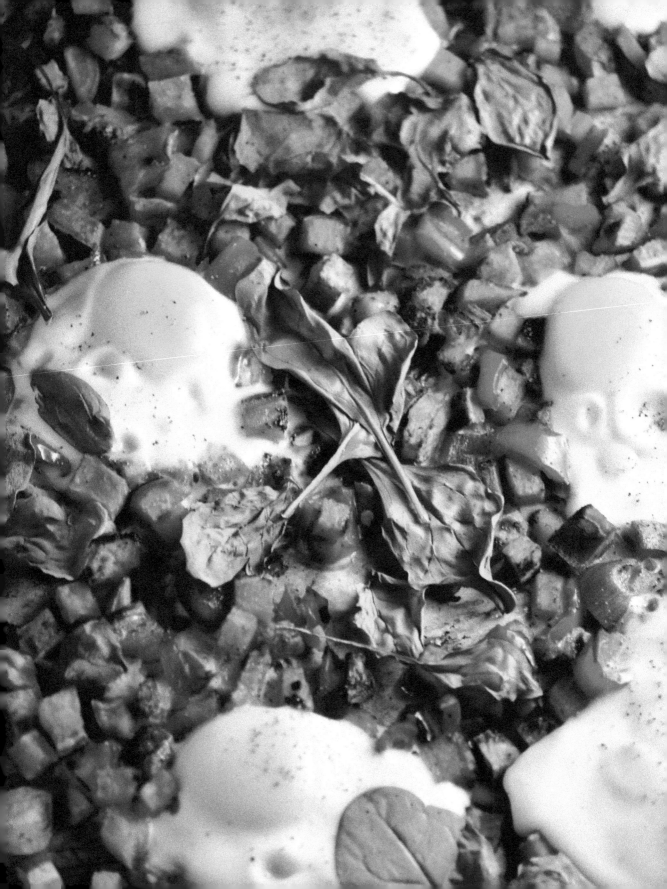

Sheet Pan Sweet Potato Hash with Baked Eggs

MAKES 4 TO 6 SERVINGS

While you could substitute regular potatoes for this dish, I like to use sweet potatoes, as they are packed with disease-fighting nutrients and have a vibrant color. This is one of those great recipes you can throw together when you need a healthy breakfast that can also pass for lunch or even an easy dinner. It all cooks on the same baking sheet for an easy, one-pan meal. If you prefer your eggs fried or poached, just cook them separately. This is delicious topped with sliced avocado and a squeeze of lime, if tolerated.

3 cups peeled and cubed sweet potatoes (about 1 large sweet potato)

3 large shallots, roughly chopped

1 red bell pepper, seeds removed and chopped

1 tablespoon olive oil

1 teaspoon paprika

1 teaspoon garlic powder

Kosher salt and freshly ground black pepper

6 large eggs

Arugula or spinach leaves for garnish (optional)

Preheat the oven to 425°F and line a large baking sheet with parchment paper.

In a large bowl, toss the sweet potatoes, shallots, and red pepper with the olive oil, paprika, garlic powder, ½ teaspoon salt, and ¼ teaspoon pepper. Spread the mixture evenly on the sheet pan and bake for about 30 minutes until light brown, tossing halfway through.

Move the vegetables around on the sheet pan to create six cavities for the eggs, spaced out over the pan. Crack one egg into each cavity and return to the oven. Bake until the whites are just cooked through, 4 to 5 minutes. The yolks should still be soft. (The yolks will look runny even when they're cooked through, so be careful not to overcook them). If desired, garnish with arugula or spinach leaves for a little color.

To serve, using a large spatula, divide the vegetables and eggs among serving plates. Serve warm.

Baked Cinnamon Apple Oatmeal

MAKES 6 SERVINGS

The Mediterranean offers some wonderful apple dishes, whether in cakes or as baked apples. I wanted to use those same flavors in a dish that was easy to meal prep for a busy week, or to have on hand for bad days. A 2020 study showed that cinnamon could be effective for migraine prevention and to relieve pain; this recipe is a great way to use it! Feel free to add in fresh ginger as well, or completely substitute one for the other. This is a great recipe for migraine days that come with nausea—it's filling without being too heavy.

Oil or butter

¾ cup shredded sweet apple like Honeycrisp, plus 1 apple for slicing

2 large eggs

1 cup milk

¾ cup unsweetened applesauce

¼ cup honey or maple syrup

1 tablespoon vanilla extract

1 teaspoon ground cinnamon

¼ teaspoon ground nutmeg

2 teaspoons baking powder

¼ teaspoon sea salt

2 cups rolled oats

Preheat the oven to 350°F. Grease an 8-inch square baking dish with oil or butter.

In a large bowl, whisk together the shredded apple, eggs, milk, applesauce, honey or maple syrup, vanilla, cinnamon, and nutmeg until smooth. Add the baking powder, salt, and oats, stirring until blended. Pour the mixture into the prepared dish.

Thinly slice the remaining apple and layer it on top of the oat mixture. Bake until cooked through, 35 to 45 minutes. Let cool for 10 to 15 minutes.

Cut the baked oatmeal into slices to serve.

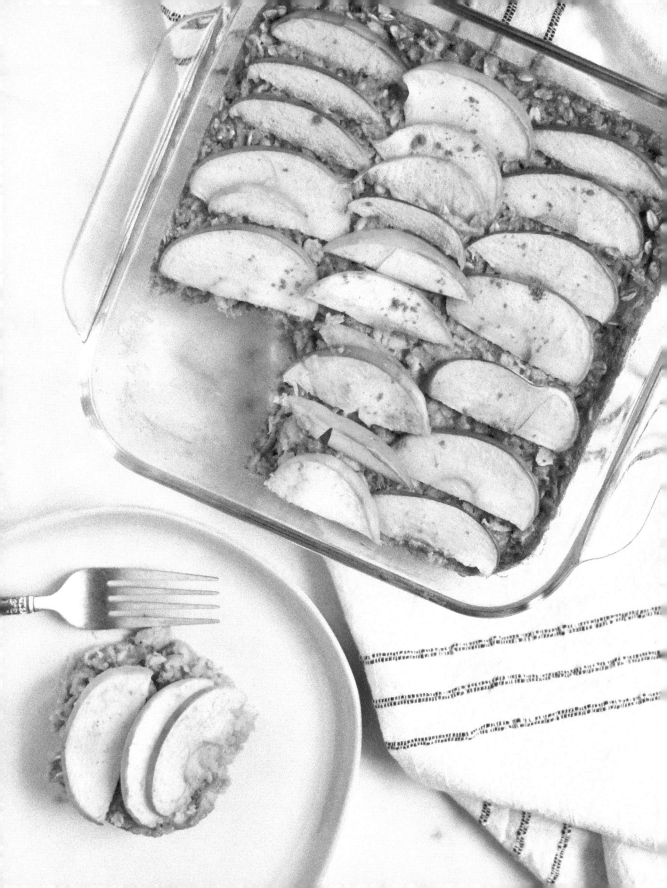

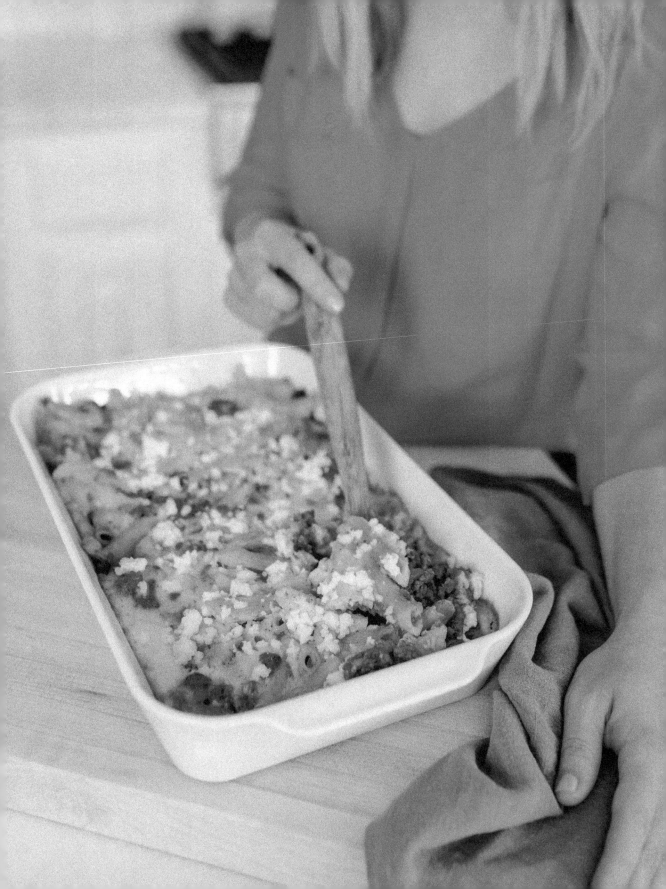

RED MEAT

THE BENEFITS OF RED MEAT

As discussed earlier, one of the characteristics of the Mediterranean diet is the low saturated fat content, which is directly related to a low consumption of red meat. But that does not mean you cannot eat any red meat while on the Mediterranean diet—consuming up to 18 ounces of lean red meat per week is acceptable. Red meat has health benefits: It is a rich source of B12, iron, zinc, and coenzyme-Q10, which are known to help with migraine control.

BEEF has been an important protein source since prehistoric times. Leaner cuts include sirloin and flank steak, but more marbled cuts have more flavor and can be eaten in moderation. When using ground beef, be sure to select products that are at least 90% lean.

BISON has a lighter flavor compared to beef. It is leaner, with a lower fat and saturated fat content than beef. Bison also has a higher iron and protein content. As such, bison may be a great substitute for beef if you are looking for a meat with low saturated fat content.

LAMB is often used in Mediterranean cuisine. Lamb refers to the meat of sheep in its first year. Lamb is a unique red meat because it contains more medium-chain fatty acids (which are less atherogenic—promoting plaque in the arteries—compared to long-chain fatty acids) and conjugated linolenic acid (which can reduce body fat) compared to beef.

SHOPPING FOR RED MEAT

There are a few ways to shop for beef. Unlike chicken or turkey, fresh beef generally doesn't have the risk of hidden additives or fillers. However, it is important to take into consideration if it is flavored or marinated. Buying pure beef and then marinating it at home is the best bet for a migraine-friendly diet.

Local butchers generally have the freshest meat in quality cuts. If you have no idea how to pick out a good cut of meat, they are typically happy to assist. Don't be shy—tell them what you are cooking and ask them for advice on choosing the right cut. Becoming friends with the local butcher can often yield amazing benefits.

Fresh beef is typically very vibrant in color and turns a grey-brown as it ages. For steaks, don't avoid fat! Look for even marbling throughout the steak rather than large fatty sections, or no fat at all. This will give you the best flavor.

For grilling, I generally like to go with filets or New York strip—these don't need a marinade and they're good to go simply grilled. Tougher cuts, like flank or skirt steak, are less expensive, but do require a marinade to help break down the fibers and make it more tender. One thing to be careful of is marinating too long, which can make the meat mushy as the fibers break down too much. Avoid marinating longer than 24 hours before you plan to cook.

Boneless beef chuck roast is also a tough cut but has really wonderful flavor. Because of these factors, low and slow cooking is a great way to get it nice and tender, while taking advantage of its great flavor. It is perfect for stew meat, pot roast, or shredded beef tacos.

Lamb is one of my favorite types of meat. It is so flavorful, especially paired with Mediterranean flavors like rosemary, garlic, and even cinnamon! Don't let the cinnamon deter you—it takes average ground beef or lamb dishes to the next level in flavor. I chose ground lamb for these recipes as I believe it's the easiest to locate in most grocery stores (or easy to substitute beef if you cannot). But if you want to branch out, try some of the Basil Garlic Aioli (page 219) with a simply roasted rack of lamb, or seared lamb chops.

Much like fish, if access to a local butcher or fresh cuts of meat isn't an option, delivery packages like ButcherBox are a good backup option.

Easy Pastitsio Bake

MAKES 6 SERVINGS

This recipe is a Greek-style version of my grandma's recipe for Lazy Lasagna—a family favorite. Pastitsio has many of the same elements as a lasagna—a creamy white béchamel sauce, and long pasta tubes featuring cinnamon-scented ground lamb and feta cheese. To make this easy, I used penne and cut out the usual fancy layering. This is a good choice to make ahead or to give to a friend in need. If you prefer ground beef over lamb, look for beef with 85/15 fat content for best results.

Kosher salt and freshly ground black pepper

10 ounces whole-wheat pasta shells or penne rigate

1 pound ground lamb

1 tablespoon olive oil, plus more for cooking

2 large shallots, chopped (about ½ cup)

2 garlic cloves, minced

¼ cup tomato paste

½ teaspoon cinnamon

BÉCHAMEL SAUCE

⅓ cup extra-virgin olive oil

⅓ cup all-purpose flour

2¾ cups milk

¼ teaspoon ground nutmeg

Kosher salt and freshly ground black pepper

4 ounces fresh feta cheese (packed in water)

Preheat the oven to 350°F. Oil a 9-by-13-inch baking pan.

Bring a large pot of salted water to a boil over high heat. When the water comes to a boil, cook the pasta according to package directions. Drain through a colander and set aside.

In a large skillet over medium heat, add the ground lamb, breaking it up into small pieces with a wooden spoon. Season with ½ teaspoon salt and ¼ teaspoon black pepper, and cook until no longer pink, about 5 minutes. Transfer the meat to a paper towel-lined plate to drain the excess oil. Wipe out the pan.

In the same pan, still over medium heat, warm the olive oil. Add the shallots and cook, stirring often, until softened, 1 to 2 minutes. Add the garlic, tomato paste, and cinnamon and stir until well blended and fragrant, about 5 minutes. Reduce the heat to low and mix in the cooked lamb.

To make the Béchamel Sauce, in a large saucepan over medium heat, warm the oil. Whisk in the flour until smooth. Let the flour mixture bubble and turn a light brown color, 1 to 2 minutes. Reduce the heat to low and add the milk about ¼ cup at a time, whisking until smooth before adding each addition. Increase the heat to medium and cook, stirring often, as it begins to simmer (small bubbles). Allow the sauce to bubble and thicken until the sauce leaves a line on the bottom of the pan when you run a wooden spoon across it, about 5 minutes. Stir in the nutmeg and salt and pepper to taste.

CONTINUED ON PAGE 211

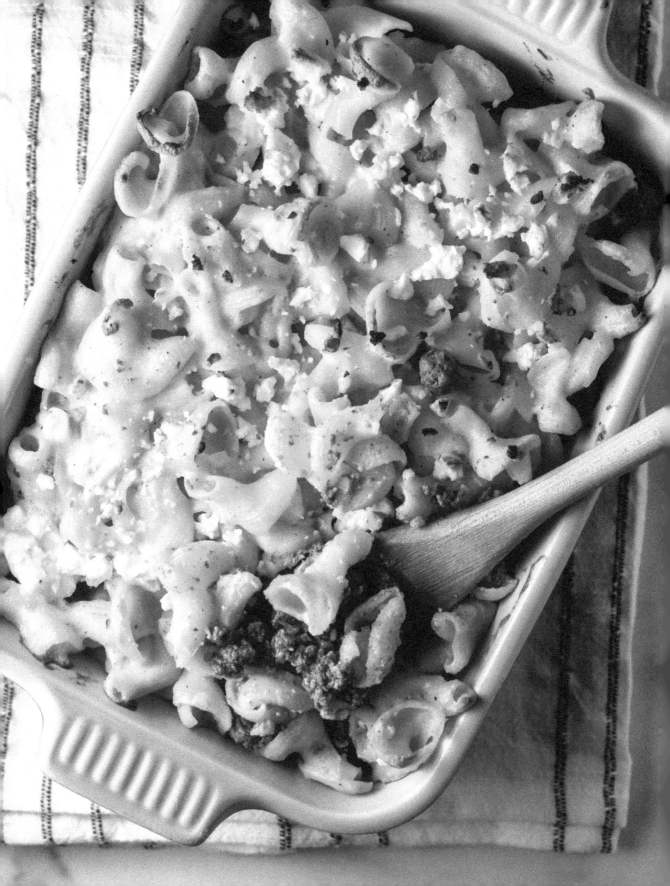

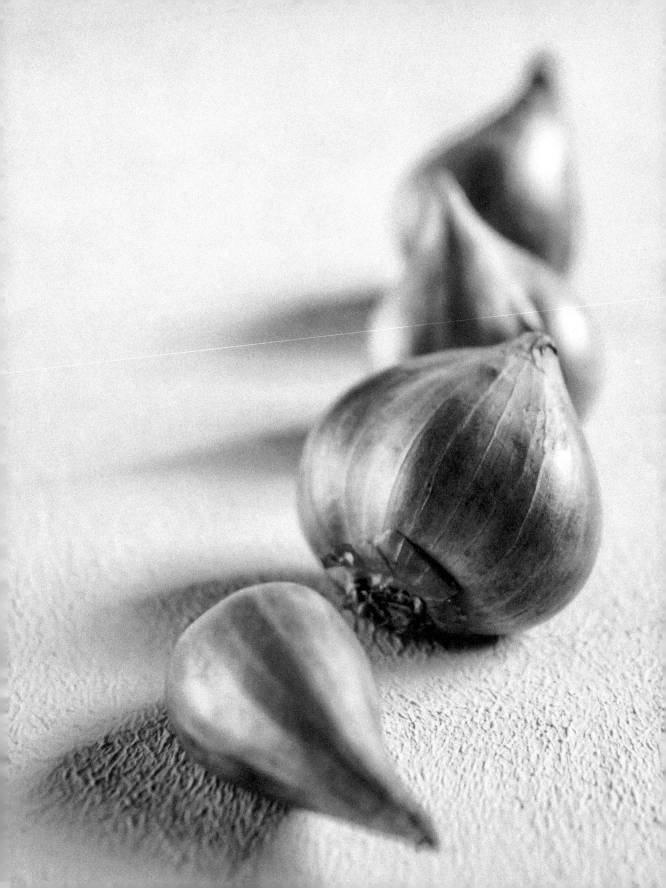

Easy Pastitsio Bake (continued)

Stir the pasta into the béchamel sauce until well coated. Add half of the pasta to the prepared pan and spread out evenly. Top the pasta with the lamb mixture. Top with the remaining pasta and spread out evenly. Sprinkle the crumbled feta cheese on top. Bake until bubbling and lightly browned on top, 25 to 30 minutes.

Remove the pastitsio from the oven and let cool slightly. Use a large spoon to divide it among serving plates. Serve warm.

NOTE: For a dairy-free dish, use oat milk instead of dairy milk and omit the feta cheese. For a gluten-free dish, use gluten-free pasta and substitute 2 tablespoons cornstarch or arrowroot powder in the béchamel sauce.

TIP: For a lower sodium alternative, replace the feta cheese with crumbled goat cheese.

Pomegranate Beef & Vegetable Skewers

MAKES 4 TO 6 SERVINGS

In this recipe, pomegranate molasses (concentrated pomegranate juice), pairs surprisingly well with grilled beef in these easy-to-make beef and vegetable skewers. Pomegranate molasses can be found at health food stores or online, but it is also easy to make at home by simply reducing pomegranate juice until it becomes thick and syrupy. You'll need wooden or metal skewers to make this dish.

3 garlic cloves, minced

3 tablespoons extra-virgin olive oil

2 tablespoons pomegranate molasses

1 tablespoon distilled white vinegar

1 tablespoon honey

½ teaspoon kosher salt

Freshly ground black pepper

2 pounds sirloin or New York strip steak, cut into 1- to 1½-inch cubes

2 bell peppers (red, yellow, or green), cut into bite-size chunks

3 to 4 large shallots, cut into bite-size chunks

8 ounces white button mushrooms, wiped clean

Chopped fresh parsley for garnish

In a large bowl, mix together the garlic, olive oil, pomegranate molasses, vinegar, honey, salt, and a few grinds of pepper. Add the steak cubes and stir until well coated. Cover and marinate the steak in the refrigerator for at least 1 hour and up to 24 hours. The longer the steak marinates, the stronger the pomegranate flavor will be. (I like to marinate for 6 to 7 hours.)

Remove the steak from the refrigerator and let it stand at room temperature at least 15 minutes before cooking. If you're using wooden skewers, soak them in water while the steak is warming.

Preheat a gas or charcoal grill to medium-high heat, 400° to 450°F. Onto metal or soaked wooden skewers, thread the meat, bell peppers, shallots, and mushrooms in an alternating pattern and set on a plate.

When the grill is hot, place the skewers on the grill at an angle and close the lid. Grill, turning the skewers every 2 to 3 minutes, turning about 3 times total, until the beef is lightly charred on the outside, about 6 minutes for medium (145°F), or until cooked to your liking.

Transfer the skewers to a large plate, cover with foil, and let rest for 5 minutes. To serve, divide the skewers among serving plates and serve warm.

TIP: If the steak at the butcher counter seems very fatty, increase the amount to 2½ pounds and trim the excess fat before cutting it into cubes.

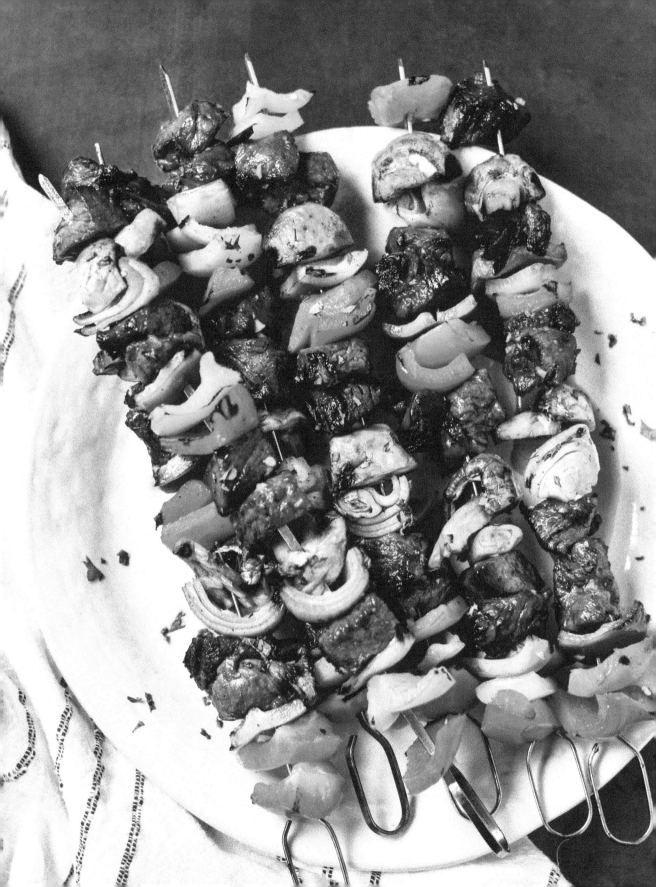

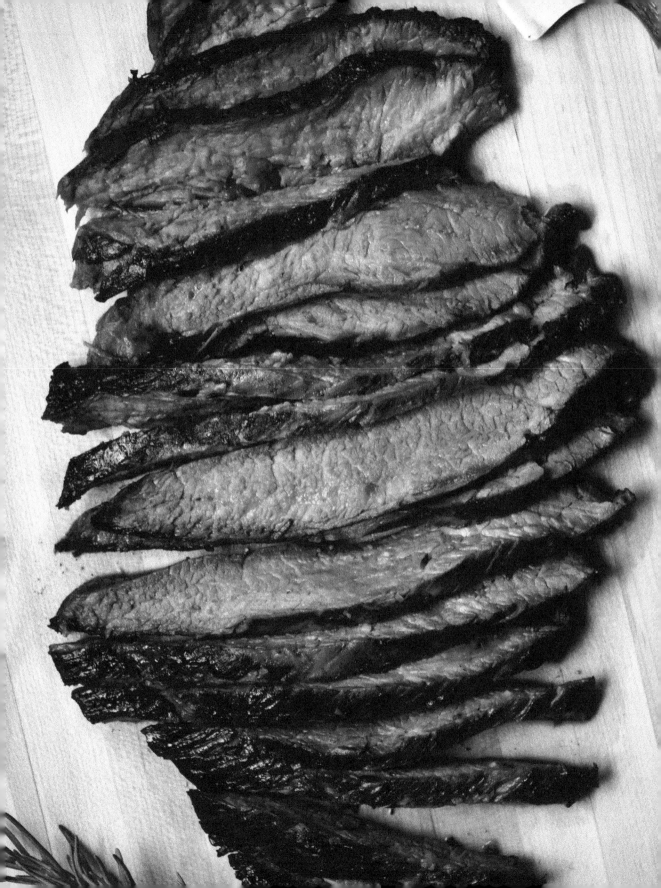

Tart Cherry Grilled Steak

MAKES 4 SERVINGS

This is a staple in our house, and tart cherry juice contains so many wonderful benefits for migraine that it's helpful to sneak it into recipes wherever you can. It takes very little prep time, but you have to plan ahead a bit so that the steak has time to marinate. Another benefit is that there are no dirty dishes except tongs, a chef's knife, and a cutting board… what is this magic?!

Tart Cherry Marinade
  (page 48)
2½ pounds flank steak
Olive oil spray

Prepare the tart cherry marinade and place it in a shallow bowl with the flank steak. Cover and refrigerate for at least 2 hours up to 24 hours. The flavor will intensify the longer the steak marinates.

Remove the steak from the refrigerator and let stand at room temperature at least 15 minutes before cooking.

Preheat a gas or charcoal grill or a grill pan to high heat. Grease the grill grates or grill pan with oil.

When you're ready to cook, reduce the heat to medium-high. Remove the steak from the marinade and place it on the grill or grill pan. Cook until pronounced grill marks appear on the bottom of the meat, 6 to 8 minutes. Turn the meat over and cook until a meat thermometer inserted in the center registers 145°F for medium, 5 to 6 minutes, or until cooked to your liking. Transfer the steak to a carving board and cover with foil. Allow it to rest for 10 minutes.

To serve, using a long, sharp knife, slice the steak thinly against the grain (in the opposite direction of where the fibers are running) and serve warm.

Slow Cooker Braised Beef

MAKES 4 TO 6 SERVINGS

Here's another great make-ahead meal, one that basically saved me in my postpartum haze when I could barely find time to eat… much less cook. You just throw everything into a slow cooker and wait a few hours for a delicious and hearty meal. Serve over simple mashed potatoes, cauliflower, or Whipped Parsnips from *The Dizzy Cook* cookbook (page 183). If you want a faster dish, brown the meat in a large Dutch oven, then add the remaining ingredients and cook in a preheated 325°F oven for 3 to 4 hours. Sometimes it's difficult to find a large boneless chuck roast; two pieces of chuck that are 2 to 2½ pounds works well, too.

One 3- to 4-pound boneless beef chuck roast, trimmed of excess fat

2 tablespoons olive oil

Kosher salt and freshly ground black pepper

12 ounces (about 6) large carrots, peeled and cut into 2- to 3-inch chunks

4 to 5 Yukon gold potatoes, cut into 2- to 3-inch chunks

3 shallots, sliced

2 garlic cloves, minced

¾ cup tart cherry juice

¼ cup distilled white vinegar

2 cups broth or stock of choice

2 to 3 sprigs each fresh thyme and rosemary

1 bay leaf

Take the roast out of the refrigerator about 30 minutes before you start cooking.

In a large skillet, warm the oil over medium-high heat until hot, but not smoking. Season meat with salt and pepper on all sides. Add the meat to the pan and sear until golden brown on all sides, 6 to 7 minutes per side. Transfer the meat to a slow cooker. Add carrots, potatoes, shallots, garlic, tart cherry juice, vinegar, broth, thyme, rosemary, and bay leaf.

Following the manufacturer's instructions, slow-cook the meat and vegetables on the low setting until the meat falls apart easily, 8 to 9 hours. Cooking too quickly on high heat can result in tough meat.

Carefully transfer the beef to a serving dish, avoiding any excess fat. The potatoes can be placed in a separate bowl and mashed using a potato masher or fork; or just serve them whole. Arrange the shallots and carrots in the dish with the beef and potatoes. Spoon a little bit of the pan juices over the top and serve right away.

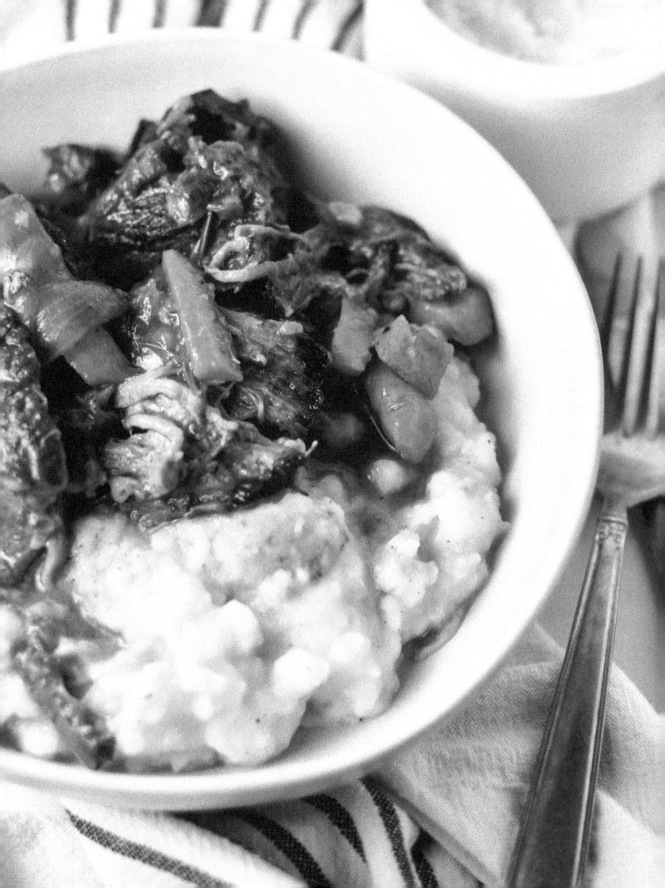

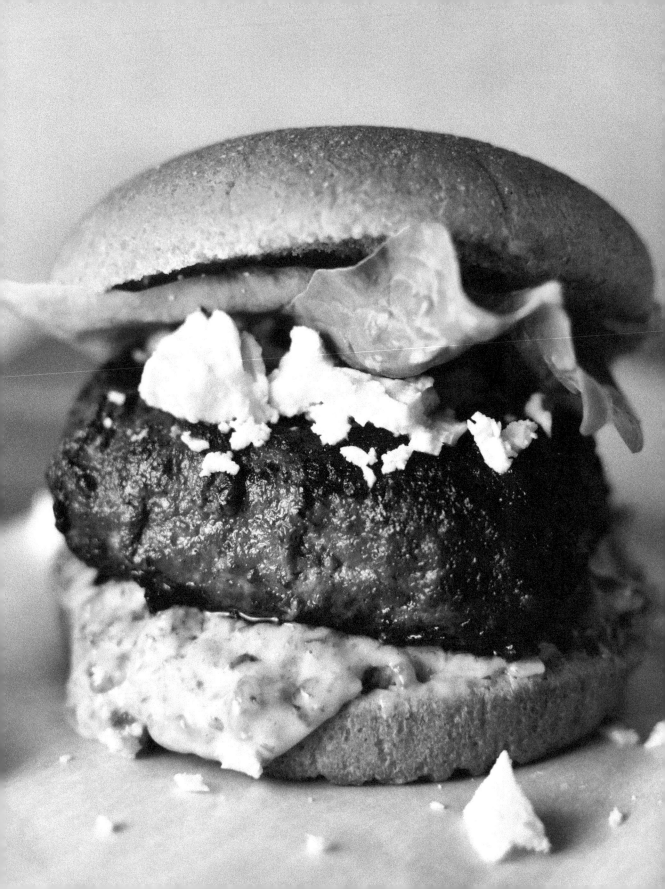

Lamb Burgers with Basil Garlic Aioli

MAKES 4 SERVINGS

Burgers happen at least one night a week in our house because they are so quick and easy. Ground lamb is easy to store in the freezer for a few months and defrost as needed. This recipe works with ground lamb or bison, and lean ground beef. You can also substitute goat cheese for the feta if you like, or need a low sodium option. The basil garlic aioli is so good and is also perfect for dipping roasted potato wedges, which I recommend serving with this. If sensitive to tomatoes, the aioli is still delicious if you omit them.

BASIL GARLIC AIOLI
½ cup mayonnaise

1 or 2 garlic cloves

2 tablespoons roughly chopped fresh basil

1 tablespoon chopped sun-dried tomatoes

¼ teaspoon freshly ground black pepper

BURGERS
2 pounds ground lamb or bison

Kosher salt and freshly ground black pepper

4 whole-wheat burger buns

Fresh spinach

½ cup crumbled feta cheese

To make the aioli, in a small food processor, combine the mayonnaise, garlic, basil, sun-dried tomatoes, and pepper. Pulse until well blended and set aside.

To make the burgers, take the meat out of the refrigerator at least 15 minutes before you start cooking.

Preheat a gas or charcoal grill to medium-high heat, 400° to 450°F. Divide the meat into four ½-pound portions. You can use your hands to form the patties, but the warmth of your hands melts the fat and can cause overworked meat if handled too much. Instead, try pressing the meat between two flat plastic lids or paper plates. I've found this results in the juiciest burgers!

Season the patties with salt and pepper just before grilling. Seasoning them too early will draw out moisture and result in a tougher burger. Place the patties on the grill and cook for about 4 to 5 minutes per side for medium, or until cooked to your liking. Transfer the patties to a plate and cover with foil. Allow them to rest for 5 to 10 minutes.

To assemble, spread the aioli on the bottom buns, then top each with a lamb patty. Top with the spinach and cheese and cover with the top buns. Serve right away.

NOTE: For a dairy-free dish, omit the feta cheese. For a gluten-free dish, substitute your favorite gluten-free bun or serve the patties atop mixed greens.

Best Recipes to Make Ahead

Decrease your stress levels with these easy recipes that will aid you through a busy work week. Double the recipe and batch-cook for several meals.

- Anti-Inflammatory Chia Pudding, page 60
- Quick Seed Granola, page 63
- Garbanzo, Shallot & Chard Salad, page 71 (add a jammy egg on top or grilled meat)
- Boursin Broccoli Soup, page 84
- Tahini Sweet Potato Bowl, page 83
- Nomato Sauce, page 96
- Sweet Potato & Grain Salad with Parsley Vinaigrette, page 102
- Couscous & Lamb Stuffed Peppers, page 105
- Turmeric-Ginger Rice, page 106
- Spinach Orzo Pasta Salad, page 109 (keep the dressing separate and mix together before serving for best flavors)
- One-Pot Creamy Mac & Cheese, page 117
- Creamy White Bean & Kale Soup, page 126
- Hearty Lentil Soup, page 129
- Mozzarella Tuna Melts, page 157 (make tuna ahead and apply to bread before serving)
- Pan-Seared Salmon with Warm Lentil Salad, page 162

- Salmon Salad Quinoa Bowl, page 165 (keep everything separate and mix together before eating to avoid soggy lettuce)
- Coastal Chicken Salad, page 172
- Chicken & Artichoke Casserole, page 180
- Chicken Meatballs with Creamy Spinach Sauce, page 183
- Rosemary Chicken & Rice Casserole, page 184
- Broccoli Artichoke Quiche Cups, page 194
- Super-Easy Egg Casserole, page 197
- Tarragon Egg Salad, page 198
- Sheet Pan Sweet Potato Hash, page 201 (keep eggs separate and pan-fry them before serving)
- Baked Cinnamon Apple Oatmeal, page 202
- Easy Pastitsio Bake, page 208
- Pomegranate Beef & Vegetable Skewers, page 212
- Slow Cooker Braised Beef, page 217
- Lamb Burgers with Basil Garlic Aioli, page 219 (assemble before serving)

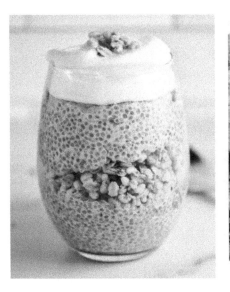
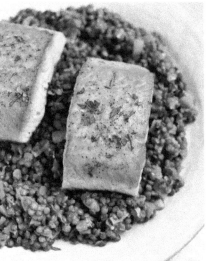
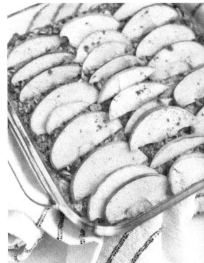

Best Dishes to Freeze

These are great recipes to make ahead on good days and store in the fridge. Often, I plan these for medical procedures, busy work weeks, or friends who just had a baby or are going through hard times. The braised beef, pastitsio bake, soups, and cookies are my favorites to give to friends and family in need.

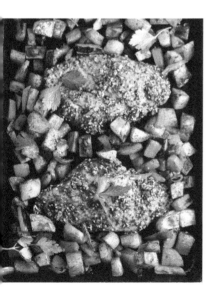
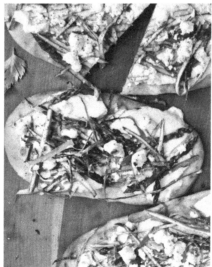
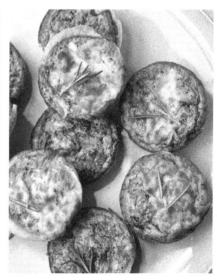

Migraine-Friendly Menus

Planning meals ahead of time is always helpful, but it is particularly so when you are dealing with a health condition, such as migraine. Here are some ideas for pairing dishes to take some of the guess-work out of meal planning.

BUSY WEEK MEAL PLAN
Prep these on Sunday and meal preparation will be effortless.

BREAKFAST
- Baked Cinnamon Apple Oatmeal (page 202)

LUNCH
- Creamy White Bean & Kale Soup (page 126)
- Coastal Chicken Salad (page 172)

DINNER
- Za'atar Roast Chicken with Sumac Potatoes & Carrots (page 175)
- Tahini Sweet Potato Bowl (page 83)

HIGH PAIN OR DIZZY DAY RECIPES
These recipes are packed with symptom-soothing ingredients, have minimal prep work, or make great comfort food. (*Good for high-nausea days.)

- Famous Migraine-Fighting Smoothie* (page 76)
- Pumpkin Seed Smoothie (page 56)
- Anti-Inflammatory Chia Pudding* (page 60)
- Rustic Toasts with Shaved Vegetables & Whipped Goat Cheese (page 110)
- Hearty Lentil Soup (page 129)
- One-Pot Creamy Broccoli Mac & Cheese (page 117)
- Mozzarella Tuna Melts (page 157)
- Turmeric-Ginger Rice* (page 106)

DATE NIGHT DINNERS
Special nights at home really helped me and my husband connect while going through a tough diagnosis. Cooking with your partner can be a wonderful experience, especially when you try new recipes together.

STARTER
- Berry, Beet & Goat Cheese Salad (page 40)

MAIN COURSE
- Seared Scallops with Vegetable Ragout (page 146) or Baked Halibut & Goat Cheese Pasta (page 161)

DESSERT
- Vanilla Honey Pudding with Fresh Berries (page 39)

OUTDOOR SUMMER DINNER
Served with a refreshing pear mocktail (see thedizzycook.com), these easy dishes are great for a potluck or summer barbecue.

- Artichoke Hummus (page 125)
- Melon & Basil Salad (page 44)
- Spinach Orzo Salad (page 109)
- Siesta Salad (page 122)
- Open-Face Fish Salad Sandwich (page 154)

STRETCH YOUR COOKING SKILLS & PALATE

The recipes below are a little more adventurous with both flavors and cooking skills. You'll feel so accomplished after making them. (Please tag #thedizzycook if you share them on social media!)

- Roasted Cauliflower & Saffron Pasta (page 114)
- Roasted Olive Chicken with Couscous (page 187)
- Seared Duck with Cherry Sauce (page 188)
- Patatas Bravas with Cod & Crispy Kale (page 142)
- Whole Roasted Branzino with Fresh Herbs (page 158)
- Easy Pastitsio Bake (page 208)

DISHES KIDS WILL LOVE

These are a few recipes that my 15-month-old son can't get enough of. The pomegranate beef skewers are his ultimate favorite.

- Boursin Broccoli Soup (page 84)
- Ricotta Kale Fritters (page 68)
- One-Pot Creamy Broccoli Mac & Cheese (page 117)
- Easy Air-Fried Falafels (page 130)
- Chicken Meatballs with Creamy Spinach Sauce (page 183)
- Pomegranate Beef & Vegetable Skewers (page 212)
- Slow Cooker Braised Beef (page 216)
- Lamb Burgers with Basil Garlic Aioli (page 219)

HOLIDAY MEALS

Here are a handful of recipes worthy of any special occasion meal.

BREAKFAST

- Super-Easy Egg Casserole (page 197) or Broccoli Artichoke Quiche Cups (page 194)

STARTER

- Berry, Beet & Goat Cheese Salad (page 40)

MAIN DISHES

- Pan-Seared Salmon with Warm Lentil Salad (page 162)
- Slow Cooker Braised Beef (page 216)
- Seared Duck with Cherry Sauce (page 188)

SIDE DISHES

- Garlicky Roasted Green Beans (page 88)
- Whipped Parsnips (page 183 of *The Dizzy Cook* cookbook)

DRINK

- Tart Cherry Nightcap (page 47)

COZY MEDITERRANEAN-STYLE DINNER

If you're in the mood for a comforting meal, these dishes go particularly well together.

MAIN COURSE

- Rosemary Chicken & Rice Casserole (page 184) or Chicken and Artichoke Casserole (page 180)

SIDE DISH

- Za'atar Roasted Carrots (page 87)

DESSERT

- Honey Tahini Cookies (page 59)

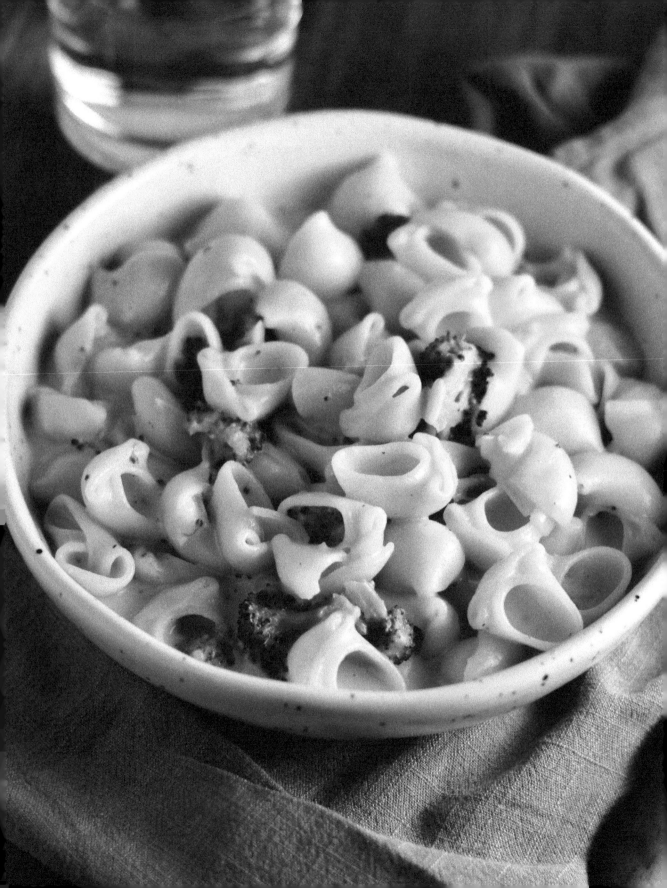

References

De Filippis F, Pellegrini N, Vannini L, et al. High-level adherence to a Mediterranean diet beneficially impacts the gut microbiota and associated metabolome. Gut 2016;65:1812-1821

Jaacks L.M., Sher S., Staercke C., Porkert M., Alexander W.R., Jones D.P., Vaccarino V., Ziegler T.R., Quyyumi A.A. Pilot randomized controlled trial of a Mediterranean diet or diet supplemented with fish oil, walnuts, and grape juice in overweight or obese US adults. BMC Nutr. 2018;4:2639

Jennings A., Berendsen A.M., de Groot L.C.P.G.M., Feskens E.J.M., Brzozowska A., Sicinska E., Pietruszka B., Meunier N., Caumon E., Malpuech-Brugère C., et al. Mediterranean-Style Diet Improves Systolic Blood Pressure and Arterial Stiffness in Older Adults. Hypertension. 2019;73:578–586

Keys A, Menotti A, Karvonen MJ, et al. The diet and 15-year death rate in the seven countries study. Am J Epidemiol 1986;124:903-915.

Martinez-Huelamo M, Vallverdu-Queralt A, Di Lecce G, et al. Bioavailability of tomato polyphenols is enhanced by processing and fat addition: evidence from a randomized feeding trial. Mol Nutr Food Res 2016;60(7):1578-1589

Meslier V., Laiola M., Roager H.M., De Filippis F., Roume H., Quinquis B., Giacco R., Mennella I., Ferracane R., Pons N., et al. Mediterranean diet intervention in overweight and obese subjects lowers plasma cholesterol and causes changes in the gut microbiome and metabolome independently of energy intake. Gut. 2020;69:1258–1268

Oruna-Concha MJ, Methven L, Blumenthal H, et al. Differences in glutamic acid and 5'-ribonucleitide contents between flesh and pulp of tomatoes and the relationship with umami taste. J Agric Food Chem 2007;55:5776-5780

Ramsden, Christopher E., et. al. Dietary alteration of n-3 and n-6 fatty acids for headache reduction in adults with migraine: randomized controlled trial. BMJ. 2021;374:n1448.

Resources

Many of these places are great ways to learn more and find support!
- The Dizzy Cook: www.thedizzycook.com
- The Dizzy Cook Recipe Chat on Facebook to help with recipe questions
- Dr. Shin Beh's Office: www.vestibularmd.com
- American Migraine Foundation: www.americanmigrainefoundation.org
- VEDA (vestibular migraine and vestibular disorders): www.vestibular.org
- Miles for Migraine: www.milesformigraine.org
- Association of Migraine Disorders: www.migrainedisorders.org
- National Headache Foundation and the Heads UP Podcast: headaches.org
- My Chronic Brain: www.mychronicbrain.com

Index

Note: Page references in *italics* indicate photographs.

Acknowledgments

I didn't think it was possible to write a cookbook while managing vestibular migraine and a newborn, but when Dr. Beh mentioned the idea I knew I couldn't turn it down. He is a big reason why I can push myself more these days, always supporting me not only in my treatment plan, but also with my career shift. I can't even begin to imagine what life might have turned out to be without his guidance, but I can guarantee I would not be in the same place. Thank you for continuing to care for both my friends and my family, making a huge difference in their lives as well.

It's a scary thing to lose who you thought you were going to be when diagnosed with vestibular migraine. When I started The Dizzy Cook, I had no idea if it would even work, and to see how much it has grown over the years has made me so happy. I want to thank the dedicated readers. You guys are the reason I keep going when I'm so tired or have days of doubt. Any time I'm feeling down, one of you sends me a message or email that lifts my spirits. You have no idea how much your support means to me, and that I save all your messages and read them on my hardest days.

Casey, while you didn't wash as many dishes this time around, you have always supported me and encouraged me. I'm able to give so much to others because you give me so much to me. And George, my littlest taste tester, you arrived at just the right time. I hope you continue to love my pastitsio and berry smoothie as much as you do right now. Mom, thank you for being the best babysitter while I worked through difficult days (and helping with those dishes). I love you all so much.

To my editor Jen, thanks for always believing in me and also handling all my last minute freak out edits. I couldn't ask for a better editor and VM friend. You always support me in my vision and I'm so lucky you found me early on!

To the WMP team: Rachel, Alice and Olivia, you guys are rockstars! Thanks for always doing a wonderful job, being super flexible when I change my mind about photos a million times, and bringing our writing to life.

Friends and family—you are my favorite people to cook for and we are so thankful for your help with George while our lives got a little chaotic. Thanks for always making my recipes and sharing them with others even when you don't live with a migraine disorder!

A big thank you to Angie Garcia for filling in with some beautiful photos and making Dr. Beh and myself look great. Amy, Toby, and Elizabeth—thank you so much for inspiring others with what you cook up at home and helping me with recipe chat. You guys are seriously the best (and help me to bless and release!). To my VEDA team as well as my very first VM friend, Kayla—thanks for being there for me from the beginning!

I also want to honor Association of Migraine Disorders, American Migraine Foundation, Miles for Migraine, CHAMP and Retreat Migraine, Migraine Meanderings, National Headache Foundation, My Chronic Brain and Migraine Again for giving me a platform to use my talents to help others in the kitchen. Nothing brings me more joy than helping others with migraine find comfort and good days through cooking. —Alicia Wolf

It truly takes a team to bring such a project to fruition. My utmost gratitude and appreciation goes to Yessie, my rock, my muse, and my right hand, for always being there for me and helping me realize this work. I would not be where I am today without you. Special thanks to Alicia Wolf, whose creative prowess was the driving force of this book; your advocacy and energy is amazing. A big thank you to my family, for supporting me. Finally, much appreciation to Jennifer Newens and the fantastic team at West Margin Press for keeping me on schedule, editing and helping us produce this wonderful book.—Shin Beh, MD, FAAN, FAHS

VOLUME EQUIVALENTS (LIQUID)

US Standard	US Standard (Ounces)	Metric
2 tablespoons	1 fl. oz.	30 mL
¼ cup	2 fl. oz.	60 mL
½ cup	4 fl. oz.	120 mL
1 cup	8 fl. oz.	240 mL
1½ cups	12 fl. oz.	355 mL
2 cups or 1 pint	16 fl. oz.	475 mL
4 cups or 1 quart	32 fl. oz.	1 L

OVEN TEMPERATURES

Fahrenheit (F)	Celsius (C)
250	120
300	150
325	165
350	180
375	190
400	200
425	220
450	230

VOLUME EQUIVALENTS (DRY)

US Standard	Metric (Approximate)
⅛ teaspoon	.5 mL
¼ teaspoon	1 mL
½ teaspoon	2 mL
¾ teaspoon	4 mL
1 teaspoon	5 mL
1 tablespoon	15 mL
¼ cup	59 mL
⅓ cup	79 mL
½ cup	118 mL
⅔ cup	156 mL
¾ cup	177 mL
1 cup	235 mL
2 cups or 1 pint	475 mL
3 cups	700 mL
4 cups or 1 quart	1 L
½ gallon	2 L

WEIGHT EQUIVALENTS

US Standard	Metric
½ ounce	15 g
1 ounce	30 g
2 ounces	60 g
4 ounces	115 g
8 ounces	225 g
12 ounces	340 g

ALICIA WOLF is the author of *The Dizzy Cook* cookbook and the voice behind thedizzycook.com, an award-winning blog dedicated to improving the diet and lifestyle for those who suffer from migraine. She works with the Vestibular Disorders Association and Miles for Migraine, and has been featured on the Association of Migraine Disorders, the American Migraine Foundation, Good Morning Texas, foodgawker, National Headache Foundation, Healthline, and more. She is also a partner to the American Migraine Foundation. Alicia lives in Dallas, Texas.

SHIN C. BEH, MD, FAAN, FAHS is a neurologist specializing in balance and migraine, with a focus on vestibular migraine. He set up the University of Texas Southwestern Medical Center's very first Vestibular Neuro-Visual Disorders clinic, built to help care for those with neurological disorders that cause vertigo, dizziness, and imbalance, and is the founder of the Beh Center for Vestibular & Migraine Disorders. Dr. Beh is the author of books focusing on migraine, including *Victory Over Vestibular Migraine* and *The Migraine Manual*. He lives in Frisco, Texas.